I HAVE A GUT FEELING

How The Microbiome Holds the Key to Health

Asa Eccleston Kibilski

CONTENTS

THE HIDDEN UNIVERSE WITHIN

Introducing the Microbiome: More Than Just Bacteria

Have you ever wondered what's happening inside your body, beyond the organs and systems you learned about in biology class? There's a whole universe thriving within you, a bustling metropolis of trillions of tiny organisms that collectively make up your microbiome. It's a community so vast and diverse, it rivals the number of stars in our galaxy. And it plays a far more significant role in your health than you might imagine.

Forget the old notion that germs are simply enemies to be vanquished. Your microbiome is a complex ecosystem of bacteria, viruses, fungi, and other microbes, most of which are not only harmless but essential for your well-being. These microscopic tenants reside mainly in your gut, but they also populate your skin, mouth, lungs, and even your genitals.

Think of your gut as a rainforest, teeming with life. Each species of microbe has its own unique role to play, like the different plants and animals in a jungle ecosystem. Some help you digest food, extracting nutrients that your body can't break down on its own. Others produce vitamins, regulate your immune system, and even influence your mood and behavior.

The composition of your microbiome is as unique as your fingerprint, shaped by a combination of genetics, diet, lifestyle, and environmental factors. It begins to develop at birth, influenced by your mother's microbiome and the mode of delivery (vaginal vs. cesarean). It continues to evolve throughout your life, constantly adapting to changes in your environment and habits.

A healthy, diverse microbiome is like a well-balanced ecosystem, with a variety of species working together in harmony. But when this delicate balance is disrupted, it can have far-reaching consequences for your health. An imbalance, known as dysbiosis, has been linked to a wide range of conditions, from digestive disorders and obesity to autoimmune diseases and mental health issues.

The good news is that you have the power to nurture and restore your microbiome. By making simple changes to your diet, lifestyle, and exposure to environmental factors, you can cultivate a thriving inner ecosystem that supports your health in countless ways.

In the following chapters, we'll delve deeper into the fascinating world of the microbiome, exploring its many roles in your body and mind. We'll uncover the latest scientific discoveries, bust common myths, and provide practical tips for optimizing your gut health. Get ready to embark on a journey of discovery, as we unlock the secrets of this hidden universe within you.

Your Gut: A Thriving Ecosystem of Trillions

Imagine your gut as a bustling city, teeming with trillions of inhabitants. This isn't some dystopian sci-fi scene; this is the reality happening inside you right now. Your gut, specifically your large intestine, is home to the most densely populated microbial community on Earth, known as the gut microbiota. It's a metropolis like no other, where bacteria, viruses, fungi, and other microbes coexist in a delicate balance, each with a unique role to play in your overall health.

Think of these microbes as citizens of your gut city. Some are like hard working farmers, helping to break down complex carbohydrates into simple sugars that your body can use for energy. Others are like skilled artisans, producing essential vitamins like vitamin K and B vitamins that your body can't make on its own. Some are like diligent sanitation workers, keeping harmful pathogens at bay and maintaining a healthy environment. And others are like influential politicians, communicating with your immune system and even your brain to influence your mood and behavior.

This bustling microbial city isn't just a random collection of organisms; it's a carefully orchestrated ecosystem where different species interact in complex ways. Some species compete for resources, while others cooperate to perform specific functions. This intricate web of relationships is essential for maintaining a healthy gut environment and, by extension, your overall well-being.

The diversity of your gut microbiota is key to its resilience and ability to adapt to changing conditions. Just like a city with a diverse economy is more resilient to economic shocks, a gut with a diverse microbiota is better equipped to handle challenges like dietary changes, stress, and exposure to pathogens.

But what exactly are these microbes, and where do they come from? Bacteria are the most abundant inhabitants of your gut, making up the vast majority of your gut microbiota. They come in all shapes and sizes, from rod-shaped bacilli to spiral-shaped spirochetes. But they're not the only players in this microbial metropolis. Viruses, though often associated with illness, are also part of your gut ecosystem, infecting bacteria and influencing their behavior. Fungi, like yeasts, are also present in smaller numbers, playing a role in maintaining gut health.

Your gut microbiota is not static; it's constantly evolving and adapting to changes in your diet, lifestyle, and environment. The foods you eat provide fuel for your gut microbes, influencing which species thrive and which decline. Your lifestyle choices, such as exercise, sleep, and stress management, also impact your gut health. And exposure to environmental factors, like antibiotics and pesticides, can disrupt the delicate balance of your gut ecosystem.

Understanding the dynamics of your gut microbiota is like

unlocking a secret code to your health. By learning how to nurture and support this thriving ecosystem, you can optimize your digestion, immunity, mental health, and overall well-being. In the following chapters, we'll delve deeper into the fascinating world of gut microbes, exploring their diverse roles and how you can harness their power to improve your health.

THE GUT-BRAIN AXIS: A TWO-WAY STREET

How Gut Bacteria Influence Mood and Mental Health

Have you ever experienced "butterflies" in your stomach before a big presentation, or felt a knot in your gut when you're anxious? These aren't just figures of speech; they're real sensations that illustrate the intricate connection between your gut and your brain. This connection, known as the gut-brain axis, is a two-way communication highway where your gut bacteria play a starring role in influencing your mood, emotions, and even mental health.

It might sound surprising, but your gut microbes are not just passive residents in your body; they're active participants in your mental well-being. They produce neurotransmitters, the chemical messengers that your brain uses to communicate with itself and the rest of your body. These neurotransmitters, such as serotonin, dopamine, and GABA, play a crucial role in regulating your mood, sleep, appetite, and stress response.

Serotonin, often called the "happy hormone," is primarily produced in your gut. It's involved in regulating mood, sleep, and digestion. When your gut bacteria are out of balance, your serotonin production can be disrupted, potentially contributing to mood disorders like depression and anxiety.

Dopamine, the "reward chemical," is also produced in your gut. It plays a role in motivation, pleasure, and focus. Gut bacteria can influence dopamine levels, impacting your ability to experience pleasure and motivation.

GABA, a neurotransmitter that promotes relaxation and reduces anxiety, is also produced by gut bacteria. Imbalances in gut bacteria can lead to lower GABA levels, potentially contributing to anxiety disorders.

But the influence of gut bacteria on your mental health goes beyond just neurotransmitter production. They also communicate with your brain through the vagus nerve, a major communication pathway between your gut and your brain. This vagus nerve acts like a telephone line, transmitting signals from your gut bacteria to your brain and vice versa.

These signals can influence your brain's stress response, immune function, and even the structure of your brain. Studies have shown that gut bacteria can affect the development of certain brain regions involved in mood regulation and stress response.

The gut-brain axis is a complex and dynamic system, with ongoing research uncovering new layers of its influence on our mental well-being. While the exact mechanisms are still being elucidated, the evidence suggests that gut bacteria play a significant role in shaping our emotions, behavior, and overall mental health.

By understanding the gut-brain axis, we can gain valuable insights into how to optimize our mental well-being. Nurturing a healthy gut microbiome through diet, lifestyle, and targeted interventions may offer a promising avenue for preventing and treating mood disorders, anxiety, and even more complex mental health conditions.

The Impact of Stress on Your Microbiome

Ever notice how a stressful day can leave you feeling not only mentally drained but also physically unwell? Perhaps you experience stomach cramps, indigestion, or even a bout of diarrhea. This isn't just a coincidence; it's a clear demonstration of the intimate connection between your gut and your brain, and how stress can wreak havoc on your microbiome.

Think of your gut as a canary in a coal mine, a sensitive barometer for your overall well-being. When you're stressed, your body releases a cascade of stress hormones, like cortisol, which can have a profound impact on your gut microbes. These hormones can alter the composition and diversity of your gut bacteria, favoring the growth of harmful microbes while suppressing beneficial ones. This imbalance, known as dysbiosis, can lead to a host of digestive problems, from bloating and gas to constipation and diarrhea.

But the impact of stress on your gut goes far beyond just digestive discomfort. Chronic stress can trigger inflammation in your gut, weakening the intestinal barrier and allowing harmful substances to leak into your bloodstream. This "leaky gut" phenomenon can trigger a systemic immune response, leading to inflammation throughout your body and contributing to a variety of health issues, from allergies and autoimmune diseases to mental health disorders.

Stress can also interfere with the communication between your gut and your brain. Remember that vagus nerve, the vital communication pathway between your gut and your brain? Well, stress can disrupt the signals traveling along this nerve, leading to a breakdown in communication between these two crucial organs. This can manifest as mood swings, anxiety, difficulty concentrating, and even depression.

So, how does stress affect your gut bacteria exactly? One way is by altering the environment in your gut. Stress can reduce blood flow to your intestines, making it harder for beneficial bacteria to thrive. It can also alter the pH levels in your gut, creating a more hospitable environment for harmful microbes. Additionally, stress can change the way your gut muscles contract, leading to slower transit time for food and allowing harmful bacteria to linger longer in your gut.

The good news is that you can take steps to mitigate the impact of stress on your gut health. Stress management techniques like meditation, yoga, deep breathing exercises, and spending time in nature can help to reduce stress hormone levels and restore balance to your gut microbiome. A healthy diet rich in fiber, fermented foods, and probiotics can also support a healthy gut ecosystem. And if you're struggling with chronic stress, seeking professional help from a therapist or counselor can be an invaluable resource.

Remember, your gut and your brain are constantly communicating, and this two-way street means that your gut health can significantly impact your mental well-being, and vice versa. By understanding the intricate connection between stress and your microbiome, you can take proactive steps to protect your gut health and foster a resilient mind-body connection.

YOUR SECOND BRAIN: THE ENTERIC NERVOUS SYSTEM

The Gut's Own Neural Network

You might be surprised to learn that your gut isn't just responsible for digestion; it also houses its own complex nervous system, often referred to as the "second brain." This intricate network of neurons, neurotransmitters, and support cells, known as the enteric nervous system (ENS), runs the entire length of your gastrointestinal tract, from your esophagus to your rectum. And it's far more sophisticated than you might imagine.

Think of your ENS as a mini-brain, operating independently of your central nervous system (CNS) but still maintaining a close connection through the vagus nerve. This allows your gut to communicate with your brain and vice versa, influencing everything from digestion and gut motility to mood and emotions.

Your ENS is responsible for a wide range of functions, including:

- **Controlling gut motility:** Your ENS coordinates the contractions of your gut muscles, propelling food through your digestive tract and ensuring proper digestion and absorption of nutrients.
- **Regulating blood flow:** It controls the blood flow to your gut, ensuring adequate oxygen and nutrient delivery to the cells lining your digestive tract.
- **Secreting digestive enzymes and hormones:** It stimulates the release of enzymes and hormones that are essential for breaking down food and absorbing nutrients.
- **Sensing and responding to stimuli:** Your ENS is equipped with sensory neurons that detect changes in your

gut environment, such as the presence of food, toxins, or inflammation. It then sends signals to your gut muscles and glands to respond appropriately.

- **Maintaining gut barrier integrity:** It helps to maintain the integrity of the intestinal lining, preventing harmful substances from leaking into your bloodstream.

Your ENS contains as many neurons as your spinal cord, making it a complex and sophisticated network capable of independent decision-making. This means that your gut can function autonomously, without constant input from your brain. This is why you can still digest food even when you're sleeping or unconscious.

The neurons in your ENS communicate with each other using the same neurotransmitters as your brain, including serotonin, dopamine, and GABA. This is why your gut health can have such a profound impact on your mood and mental health. When your gut bacteria are out of balance, it can disrupt the production and function of these neurotransmitters, potentially contributing to mood disorders like depression and anxiety.

The ENS is also involved in the gut-brain axis, the two-way communication highway between your gut and your brain. It sends signals to your brain about the state of your gut, influencing your mood, emotions, and even your thoughts and behaviors. For example, when you're feeling stressed, your ENS can send signals to your brain that trigger feelings of anxiety or unease.

Understanding the role of your ENS is crucial for appreciating the intricate connection between your gut and your overall health. By nurturing your gut health, you're not just supporting digestion; you're also supporting your mental well-being and overall health.

How Gut Feelings Are More Than Just Intuition

Ever gone with your gut instinct and later found out you were right? Or felt butterflies in your stomach when you're nervous? These aren't just fleeting feelings; they're real physiological responses stemming from the intricate communication between your gut and your brain. The enteric nervous system (ENS), your gut's "second brain," plays a crucial role in these gut feelings, and they're far more than just intuition.

Think of your ENS as a sophisticated sensory organ, constantly monitoring the conditions in your gut. It's tuned into the chemical composition of your food, the presence of beneficial or harmful microbes, and even the emotions you're experiencing. When it detects something significant, it sends signals to your brain, triggering a cascade of physiological and emotional responses.

These gut feelings can manifest in various ways:

- **Intuition:** That "gut instinct" you get when making a decision or facing a challenge is often a result of your ENS picking up on subtle cues that your conscious mind might miss. Your gut has a way of processing information that goes beyond logic and reason, tapping into a deeper wisdom that can guide you toward the right path.
- **Emotions:** The butterflies you feel in your stomach when you're nervous or excited are a direct result of your ENS communicating with your brain. Your gut is intimately connected to your emotional center, and the sensations you feel in your gut can reflect your emotional state.
- **Physical sensations:** When you're stressed or anxious, your ENS can trigger physical symptoms like stomach cramps, nausea, or diarrhea. This is because your gut and brain are so interconnected that emotional distress can manifest as physical discomfort.
- **Food cravings:** Those intense cravings for certain foods might not just be your taste buds talking; they could be your gut microbes sending signals to your brain. Certain microbes thrive on specific nutrients, and they can influence your food

cravings to get what they need.

These gut feelings are not just random occurrences; they're valuable signals from your body, providing you with information about your internal state and the world around you. By learning to tune into your gut feelings, you can gain valuable insights into your health, well-being, and decision-making.

But how can you distinguish between genuine gut feelings and just wishful thinking? One way is to pay attention to the physical sensations you experience. Are you feeling a sense of ease and expansion in your gut, or a tightness and contraction? These sensations can offer clues about whether a decision or situation is aligned with your true desires and needs.

Another way is to consider the context of your gut feelings. Are they consistent with your values and priorities? Do they feel authentic and aligned with your inner wisdom? By reflecting on the context of your gut feelings, you can gain a deeper understanding of their meaning and significance.

Remember, your gut feelings are not infallible. They're just one piece of the puzzle, and it's important to consider other factors when making decisions. But by learning to trust your gut and integrate its wisdom into your decision-making process, you can tap into a powerful source of guidance and intuition.

In the next chapter, we'll explore the fascinating connection between your gut and your immune system, revealing how a healthy gut microbiome can strengthen your body's defenses and protect you from illness.

THE IMMUNE SYSTEM'S BEST FRIEND

How Gut Bacteria Train and Support Immunity

Imagine your immune system as a well-trained army, equipped with a vast arsenal of weapons to defend your body against invaders like viruses, bacteria, and parasites. But where does this army receive its training and support? A surprising answer lies in your gut, where your microbiome acts as a drill sergeant, constantly educating and strengthening your immune system to keep you healthy.

Your gut, with its vast surface area and exposure to the outside world through the foods you eat, is a major battleground for your immune system. It's here that your body encounters a constant stream of foreign substances, from harmless food particles to potentially harmful pathogens. Your gut microbiome plays a crucial role in distinguishing between friend and foe, helping your immune system identify and neutralize threats while tolerating beneficial microbes and nutrients.

Think of your gut microbes as friendly sparring partners for your immune cells. They constantly interact with your immune cells, stimulating them and helping them to mature and develop. This ongoing training is essential for maintaining a robust immune response and protecting you from infections.

One way gut bacteria train your immune system is by producing metabolites, small molecules that act as chemical messengers. These metabolites can interact with your immune cells, influencing their behavior and function. Some metabolites, like short-chain fatty acids (SCFAs), have anti-inflammatory properties and can help to dampen down an overactive immune response, preventing autoimmune diseases.

Gut bacteria also help to regulate the balance of different types of immune cells. For example, they can promote the development of regulatory T cells, which help to keep the immune system in check and prevent it from attacking your own body tissues. They can also stimulate the production of antibodies, which are proteins that bind to and neutralize pathogens.

The gut microbiome also plays a crucial role in maintaining the integrity of your gut barrier, a protective lining that prevents harmful substances from leaking into your bloodstream. This barrier is composed of specialized cells held together by tight junctions. Gut bacteria produce substances that strengthen these tight junctions, helping to seal any gaps and prevent leakage.

When your gut microbiome is out of balance, your immune system can become compromised. This can lead to an increased susceptibility to infections, as well as autoimmune diseases, allergies, and inflammatory disorders. For example, studies have shown that people with inflammatory bowel disease (IBD) often have a less diverse gut microbiome, with fewer beneficial bacteria and more harmful ones.

The good news is that you can take steps to nurture a healthy gut microbiome and support your immune system. Eating a diet rich in fiber, fermented foods, and probiotics can help to foster a diverse and balanced gut ecosystem. Avoiding unnecessary antibiotics and managing stress can also help to protect your gut microbes.

By understanding the intricate relationship between your gut bacteria and your immune system, you can take proactive steps to strengthen your body's defenses and promote overall health and well-being.

The Link Between Gut Health

and Autoimmune Disease

In a healthy body, the immune system acts as a vigilant guardian, protecting against harmful invaders like viruses, bacteria, and parasites. However, in autoimmune diseases, this guardian turns rogue, mistakenly attacking the body's own tissues. It's like a well-trained army turning on its own citizens, leading to a state of chronic inflammation and damage.

Emerging research suggests that the gut microbiome, the vast community of microbes residing in your digestive tract, plays a significant role in the development and progression of autoimmune diseases. While the exact mechanisms are still being investigated, there are several compelling links that highlight the gut's influence on immune function and autoimmune disorders.

One key factor is the gut barrier, a protective lining that separates the contents of your gut from your bloodstream. This barrier acts like a gatekeeper, allowing nutrients to pass through while keeping harmful substances and microbes out. However, when the gut barrier becomes compromised, a condition known as "leaky gut," it can trigger a chain reaction that leads to autoimmune disease.

Gut microbes play a crucial role in maintaining the integrity of this barrier. They produce substances that strengthen the tight junctions between the cells lining your gut, preventing leakage. When your gut microbiome is out of balance, with fewer beneficial bacteria and more harmful ones, the gut barrier can weaken, allowing toxins and microbes to enter your bloodstream. This can trigger an immune response, leading to inflammation and, in some cases, autoimmune attacks.

Another link between gut health and autoimmune disease lies in the balance of different types of immune cells. Gut microbes help to regulate the balance between pro-inflammatory and anti-inflammatory immune cells. When this balance is disrupted, it can lead to an overactive immune response, with the immune system attacking the body's own tissues.

For example, studies have shown that people with autoimmune diseases often have lower levels of regulatory T cells, a type of immune cell that helps to dampen down inflammation and prevent autoimmune attacks. Gut microbes play a role in promoting the development of these regulatory T cells, and imbalances in the gut microbiome can lead to a deficiency of these important cells.

Furthermore, gut microbes can influence the production of antibodies, proteins that bind to and neutralize pathogens. In some autoimmune diseases, the immune system produces antibodies that mistakenly attack the body's own tissues. Research suggests that gut microbes can influence the production of these autoantibodies, potentially contributing to autoimmune disease.

The gut microbiome is a complex and dynamic ecosystem, and its relationship with autoimmune disease is still an active area of research. However, emerging evidence suggests that by nurturing a healthy gut microbiome, we may be able to reduce the risk of autoimmune disease and even manage its symptoms.

Strategies for promoting a healthy gut microbiome include eating a diet rich in fiber, fermented foods, and probiotics, avoiding unnecessary antibiotics, managing stress, and addressing any underlying digestive issues. By taking care of your gut health, you're not only supporting your digestion; you're also protecting yourself from a wide range of chronic diseases, including autoimmune disorders.

WEIGHT MANAGEMENT: IT STARTS IN THE GUT

Microbes and Metabolism: The Connection

Have you ever wondered why some people seem to effortlessly maintain a healthy weight, while others struggle despite their best efforts? The answer may lie in a surprising place: your gut. Your gut microbiome, the vast community of microbes residing in your digestive tract, plays a significant role in how your body processes food, stores fat, and regulates appetite. In other words, your gut microbes may be holding the key to weight management.

Think of your gut microbes as tiny metabolic powerhouses, working tirelessly to extract energy from the food you eat. They break down complex carbohydrates, ferment fiber, and even produce short-chain fatty acids (SCFAs), which are used by your body as a source of energy. But not all microbes are created equal. Some are more efficient at extracting energy from food than others, and this can have a direct impact on your weight.

Studies have shown that people with obesity tend to have a different gut microbiome composition compared to lean individuals. They often have fewer types of bacteria, and the types of bacteria present may be more efficient at extracting energy from food. This means that they can potentially harvest more calories from the same amount of food, leading to weight gain over time.

But it's not just about how much energy your gut microbes extract; it's also about how they influence your metabolism. Gut microbes can interact with your hormones and enzymes involved in metabolism, affecting how your body stores fat, regulates blood sugar levels, and even influences your appetite.

For example, certain gut microbes can produce short-chain fatty acids that stimulate the release of hormones like leptin and GLP-1, which help to regulate appetite and promote feelings of fullness. When your gut microbiome is out of balance, with fewer of these beneficial bacteria, you may experience increased hunger and cravings, making it more difficult to maintain a healthy weight.

Gut microbes can also influence how your body stores fat. Some microbes promote fat storage, while others help to burn fat. Studies have shown that transplanting gut microbes from obese mice into lean mice can cause the lean mice to gain weight, suggesting that gut microbes can directly influence fat accumulation.

Additionally, gut microbes play a role in regulating inflammation, a process that can contribute to weight gain and metabolic disorders like insulin resistance and type 2 diabetes. Certain microbes can promote inflammation, while others have anti-inflammatory effects. An imbalanced gut microbiome, with more pro-inflammatory microbes, can contribute to chronic low-grade inflammation, making it harder to lose weight and maintain a healthy metabolism.

Understanding the intricate connection between your gut microbes and metabolism is key to unlocking the secrets of weight management. By nurturing a healthy and diverse gut microbiome, you can optimize your metabolism, regulate your appetite, and reduce inflammation, setting the stage for successful and sustainable weight loss.

In the next part, we'll delve deeper into the fascinating relationship between gut bacteria and food cravings, exploring how these tiny microbes can influence your desires for certain foods and sabotage your weight loss efforts.

Gut Bacteria and Food Cravings: Who's Really in Charge?

Have you ever reached for a sugary treat or a bag of chips, even when you weren't hungry? Or found yourself inexplicably craving certain foods, despite your best intentions to eat healthily? These aren't just moments of weakness; they could be your gut microbes pulling the strings.

Emerging research suggests that the trillions of microbes residing in your gut can influence your food cravings, sometimes even hijacking your willpower and driving you towards specific foods that benefit them, not necessarily you. This isn't some science fiction scenario; it's a fascinating example of how these tiny organisms can exert a powerful influence on your behavior.

But how exactly do gut microbes manipulate your cravings? There are several ways:

1. **Neurotransmitter manipulation:** Gut microbes can produce neurotransmitters, the chemical messengers that your brain uses to communicate. These neurotransmitters, like dopamine and serotonin, play a crucial role in reward and pleasure pathways. By influencing the production of these neurotransmitters, gut microbes can create cravings for foods that stimulate the release of these feel-good chemicals.

2. **Hormone mimicry:** Some gut microbes can produce molecules that mimic the hormones your body uses to regulate hunger and appetite. For example, certain bacteria can produce a molecule that resembles ghrelin, the "hunger hormone." By increasing ghrelin levels, these microbes can trick your brain into thinking you're hungry, even when you're not.

3. **Taste receptor manipulation:** Gut microbes can alter the way your taste buds perceive different flavors. For example, some microbes can increase your sensitivity to sweet tastes, making sugary foods more appealing.

Others can decrease your sensitivity to bitter tastes, making healthy but slightly bitter foods like vegetables less desirable.

4. **Nutrient manipulation:** Gut microbes need specific nutrients to survive and thrive. When they're lacking a particular nutrient, they can send signals to your brain, triggering cravings for foods that contain that nutrient. For example, if your gut microbes are low on fiber, they might trigger cravings for sugary or starchy foods that they can easily ferment.

The relationship between gut microbes and food cravings is complex and multifaceted, with ongoing research uncovering new layers of this fascinating interaction. However, it's clear that our gut microbes play a more significant role in our food choices than we previously thought.

So, does this mean we're helpless puppets, controlled by our gut microbes? Not necessarily. While gut microbes can influence our cravings, we still have the power to make conscious choices about what we eat. By understanding how our gut microbes manipulate our desires, we can become more aware of their influence and make informed decisions about our food choices.

Strategies for managing food cravings include:

- **Nurturing a healthy gut microbiome:** Eating a diet rich in fiber, fermented foods, and probiotics can help to create a balanced gut ecosystem with diverse microbes.
- **Listening to your body's signals:** Pay attention to your hunger and fullness cues, and eat when you're truly hungry, not just when your gut microbes are demanding a specific food.
- **Making healthy swaps:** Instead of reaching for sugary snacks, try satisfying your sweet tooth with fruit or yogurt. If you're craving salty chips, opt for nuts or seeds instead.

- **Managing stress:** Stress can exacerbate cravings, so finding healthy ways to manage stress, like exercise, meditation, or spending time in nature, can help to reduce cravings.

By understanding the role of gut microbes in food cravings, we can empower ourselves to make healthier choices and take control of our eating habits.

THE DIGESTIVE DETECTIVE: UNLOCKING FOOD SENSITIVITIES

Microbiome Imbalances and Digestive Disorders

Have you ever eaten a meal that left you feeling bloated, gassy, or just plain uncomfortable? Or perhaps you experience regular bouts of diarrhea, constipation, or other digestive woes? While these symptoms might seem like minor inconveniences, they could be signs of a deeper issue: an imbalance in your gut microbiome.

Your gut microbiome, the vast community of microbes residing in your digestive tract, plays a crucial role in digestion. These microbes help break down food, extract nutrients, and produce essential vitamins and metabolites. When your gut microbiome is healthy and balanced, digestion runs smoothly, and you feel your best.

However, when your gut microbiome is out of whack, it can lead to a variety of digestive problems. An imbalance, known as dysbiosis, can occur due to a variety of factors, including diet, stress, medication use (especially antibiotics), infections, and environmental toxins. When dysbiosis occurs, it can disrupt the delicate ecosystem in your gut, leading to an overgrowth of harmful bacteria, a decrease in beneficial bacteria, or both.

This imbalance can trigger a cascade of events that disrupt digestion and lead to uncomfortable symptoms. For example, an overgrowth of certain bacteria can produce excess gas, causing bloating and discomfort. Other bacteria can interfere with the absorption of nutrients, leading to diarrhea or constipation. And in some cases, an imbalanced gut microbiome can trigger inflammation in the gut, leading to conditions like irritable bowel syndrome (IBS) or inflammatory bowel disease (IBD).

But how do you know if your digestive problems are linked to your gut microbiome? One clue is to pay attention to your symptoms. If you experience regular digestive discomfort after eating certain foods, it could be a sign of food sensitivity. Food sensitivities occur when your immune system reacts to a specific food, triggering inflammation in your gut.

These sensitivities can be difficult to pinpoint because they often involve delayed reactions, with symptoms appearing hours or even days after eating the offending food. This is where gut microbiome testing can be helpful. By analyzing the composition of your gut microbes, these tests can identify potential food sensitivities and help you pinpoint the culprits behind your digestive woes.

Another clue is to consider your overall gut health. If you experience frequent bloating, gas, constipation, diarrhea, or other digestive problems, it could be a sign of an underlying gut microbiome imbalance. In this case, working with a healthcare professional to address the root cause of the imbalance can help to alleviate your symptoms and restore digestive harmony.

By understanding the link between your gut microbiome and digestive health, you can take proactive steps to nurture a healthy gut ecosystem and prevent digestive problems. Eating a diet rich in fiber, fermented foods, and probiotics can help to foster a diverse and balanced gut microbiome. Avoiding processed foods, sugary drinks, and excessive alcohol can also help to maintain gut health. And if you suspect a food sensitivity, working with a healthcare professional to identify and eliminate trigger foods can provide significant relief.

Personalized Nutrition Based

on Your Gut Profile

Imagine having a personalized roadmap for your diet, a guide tailored specifically to your unique gut microbiome. It's like having a nutritional GPS, directing you towards the foods that nourish your body and steering you away from those that trigger discomfort and inflammation. This isn't science fiction; it's the future of nutrition, and it's made possible by understanding the intricate relationship between your gut microbes and the foods you eat.

Each of us has a unique gut microbiome, shaped by a combination of genetics, diet, lifestyle, and environmental factors. This means that the foods that work for one person might not work for another. What might be a healthy and nourishing food for someone with a balanced gut microbiome could trigger digestive problems or inflammation in someone with an imbalanced gut.

This is where personalized nutrition comes in. By analyzing the composition of your gut microbiome, we can gain valuable insights into how your body processes different foods. This allows us to tailor your diet to your specific needs, optimizing your nutrition for better digestion, reduced inflammation, and improved overall health.

Personalized nutrition based on your gut profile takes into account several factors:

1. **Food Sensitivities:** Gut microbiome testing can identify potential food sensitivities, which are delayed immune reactions to specific foods. By eliminating these trigger foods from your diet, you can reduce inflammation, alleviate digestive symptoms, and improve your overall well-being.

2. **Microbial Diversity:** A diverse gut microbiome is a healthy gut microbiome. Personalized nutrition can help you identify foods that promote microbial diversity,

ensuring a balanced and resilient gut ecosystem.

3. **Nutrient Needs:** Your gut microbes play a crucial role in extracting nutrients from food. Personalized nutrition can help you identify any nutrient deficiencies and recommend foods that will provide your body with the essential vitamins, minerals, and other nutrients it needs to thrive.

4. **Metabolic Profile:** Your gut microbes can influence your metabolism, affecting how your body processes carbohydrates, fats, and proteins. Personalized nutrition can take your metabolic profile into account, recommending foods that support a healthy metabolism and help you achieve your weight management goals.

But personalized nutrition isn't just about restrictions and eliminations. It's about discovering new foods that nourish your body and delight your taste buds. It's about learning how to cook and eat in a way that supports your unique gut microbiome and promotes optimal health.

With personalized nutrition, you're not just following a generic diet plan; you're embarking on a culinary adventure tailored to your individual needs. You're discovering new flavors, textures, and ingredients that you might never have tried before. And you're learning how to create delicious and satisfying meals that support your gut health and overall well-being.

The future of nutrition is personal, and it's happening right now. By embracing personalized nutrition based on your gut profile, you can unlock the secrets of your unique biology and create a diet that nourishes your body from the inside out. It's time to ditch the one-size-fits-all approach and discover the power of personalized nutrition. Your gut, and your body, will thank you.

PROBIOTICS, PREBIOTICS, AND POSTBIOTICS: A GUT HEALTH PRIMER

The Different Types of Gut-Friendly Bacteria

Imagine your gut as a bustling garden, teeming with diverse plants that all contribute to its overall health and vibrancy. In this garden, the plants are your gut microbes, and just like different plants have different roles in a garden, different microbes play unique roles in your gut ecosystem. Probiotics, prebiotics, and the lesser-known postbiotics are like the gardeners, fertilizers, and compost that nurture and support this thriving microbial community.

Probiotics are live microorganisms that, when consumed in adequate amounts, confer a health benefit on the host. In simpler terms, they're the "good" bacteria that help to balance and diversify your gut microbiome. You can find probiotics in fermented foods like yogurt, sauerkraut, kimchi, and kefir, or as dietary supplements.

But not all probiotics are created equal. Different strains of probiotics have different effects on your gut health. Some strains are better at boosting your immune system, while others are more effective at reducing inflammation or improving digestion. It's important to choose the right probiotic strain for your specific needs, based on your individual gut microbiome and health goals.

Here are some of the most common probiotic strains and their potential benefits:

- **Lactobacillus acidophilus:** This strain is found in yogurt and other fermented dairy products. It can help to improve digestion, reduce lactose intolerance symptoms, and boost the immune system.

- **Bifidobacterium bifidum:** This strain is found in breast milk and some fermented foods. It can help to promote gut barrier integrity, reduce inflammation, and improve symptoms of irritable bowel syndrome (IBS).
- **Lactobacillus rhamnosus:** This strain is often used in probiotic supplements. It can help to prevent and treat diarrhea, reduce the risk of allergies, and boost the immune system.
- **Saccharomyces boulardii:** This strain is a yeast, not a bacteria, but it's still considered a probiotic. It can help to prevent and treat diarrhea, especially traveler's diarrhea, and reduce the risk of Clostridium difficile infection.

Prebiotics, on the other hand, are non-digestible fibers that act as food for your gut microbes. They're like the fertilizer that nourishes the plants in your gut garden, promoting the growth and activity of beneficial bacteria. You can find prebiotics in foods like onions, garlic, bananas, asparagus, and whole grains.

Prebiotics work by selectively feeding the good bacteria in your gut, helping them to outcompete harmful bacteria. This can lead to a more balanced and diverse gut microbiome, which is essential for optimal health. Prebiotics also have other benefits, such as promoting regular bowel movements, reducing inflammation, and improving mineral absorption.

Postbiotics are the newest addition to the gut health lexicon. They're the byproducts of probiotic metabolism, the substances that probiotics produce as they break down food and interact with your gut environment. Think of them as the compost that enriches the soil in your gut garden, providing nutrients and other beneficial compounds that support the growth of healthy microbes.

Postbiotics have a variety of potential benefits, including reducing inflammation, boosting the immune system, and improving gut barrier function. Some studies suggest that postbiotics may even be more effective than probiotics in certain situations, as they're more stable and less likely to be broken down by stomach acid.

Understanding the different types of gut-friendly bacteria and how they interact with your body is key to optimizing your gut health. By incorporating probiotics, prebiotics, and postbiotics into your diet and lifestyle, you can create a thriving gut ecosystem that supports your overall well-being.

Choosing the Right Supplements for Your Needs

With the growing popularity of probiotics, prebiotics, and postbiotics, the supplement aisle can feel like a jungle. Countless brands, strains, and combinations promise to revolutionize your gut health, but how do you navigate this overwhelming landscape and choose the right supplements for your needs?

Before you reach for that bottle of probiotics, it's crucial to understand that not all supplements are created equal. Different strains of probiotics have different effects, and the quality and viability of the microbes can vary significantly between brands. Moreover, prebiotics and postbiotics offer unique benefits that may be better suited to your specific needs than probiotics alone.

Here's a breakdown of key factors to consider when choosing gut health supplements:

1. **Strain Specificity:** Probiotics aren't a one-size-fits-all solution. Different strains target different health concerns. For example, Lactobacillus rhamnosus GG is well-studied for its ability to prevent and treat diarrhea, while Bifidobacterium lactis has been shown to reduce anxiety and stress. Research the specific strains included in a supplement and choose those that align with your health goals.

2. **Colony Forming Units (CFUs):** CFUs indicate the number of live bacteria in a probiotic supplement. Higher CFU counts don't necessarily guarantee better results, but they do suggest a higher concentration of viable bacteria. Aim for a supplement with at least 1 billion CFUs per serving.

3. **Quality and Viability:** Not all probiotics survive the journey through your stomach acid to reach your intestines. Look for supplements that are enteric-coated or microencapsulated, as these technologies help protect the bacteria from stomach acid and ensure they reach your gut alive.

4. **Storage and Expiration Date:** Probiotics are living organisms, and their viability can be affected by storage conditions. Choose supplements that have been stored properly and haven't expired, as expired probiotics may be less effective.

5. **Prebiotics and Postbiotics:** Don't overlook the power of prebiotics and postbiotics. Prebiotics, like inulin and fructooligosaccharides (FOS), nourish the beneficial bacteria in your gut, while postbiotics offer additional benefits like reducing inflammation and supporting gut barrier function. Consider combining probiotics with prebiotics or postbiotics for a synergistic effect.

6. **Your Individual Needs:** Your gut microbiome is unique, and your supplement choices should reflect that. Consider your individual health concerns, dietary habits, and any medications you're taking. If you have specific health conditions, consult with a healthcare professional to determine the most appropriate supplements for you.

7. **Brand Reputation and Third-Party Testing:** Choose supplements from reputable brands that have been third-party tested for quality and purity. This ensures that you're getting what you pay for and that the product is free from contaminants.

Remember, supplements are not a magic bullet for gut health. A healthy diet rich in fiber, fermented foods, and whole grains is the foundation for a thriving gut microbiome. Supplements can be a helpful addition, but they should complement, not replace, a healthy lifestyle.

By understanding the different types of gut health supplements and choosing the right ones for your needs, you can take an active role in supporting your gut microbiome and optimizing your overall health.

ANTIBIOTIC ARMAGEDDON: THE MICROBIOME UNDER ATTACK

The Collateral Damage of Antibiotic Use

Antibiotics have undoubtedly revolutionized modern medicine, saving countless lives by effectively treating bacterial infections. However, like a double-edged sword, these powerful drugs also inflict collateral damage on your gut microbiome, the delicate ecosystem of trillions of microbes that reside in your digestive tract. While antibiotics may be necessary to combat harmful bacteria, their indiscriminate use can wreak havoc on your gut's delicate balance, leaving behind a trail of unintended consequences.

Imagine your gut microbiome as a vibrant rainforest, teeming with diverse species of bacteria, each playing a vital role in maintaining your health. Antibiotics, like a raging wildfire, can sweep through this rainforest, wiping out not only the harmful bacteria they target but also countless beneficial species. This collateral damage disrupts the delicate balance of your gut ecosystem, leaving it vulnerable to opportunistic pathogens and potentially triggering a cascade of health problems.

One of the most immediate consequences of antibiotic use is diarrhea. Antibiotics can disrupt the normal gut flora, leading to an overgrowth of harmful bacteria like Clostridium difficile, which can cause severe diarrhea, abdominal pain, and even life-threatening complications. Studies have shown that up to 35% of people who take antibiotics experience antibiotic-associated diarrhea, highlighting the significant impact these drugs can have on gut health.

But the effects of antibiotics extend far beyond the immediate aftermath of treatment. Research suggests that even a single course of antibiotics can significantly alter the composition of your gut microbiome, with some changes persisting for months or even years. This disruption can lead to a decrease in the diversity of your gut bacteria, making it less resilient to future challenges and increasing your susceptibility to infections and other health problems.

Antibiotics can also affect the balance of different types of bacteria in your gut. They tend to wipe out beneficial bacteria that help to keep harmful bacteria in check, potentially leading to an overgrowth of opportunistic pathogens. This can trigger a range of issues, from digestive problems like bloating, gas, and constipation to more serious conditions like inflammatory bowel disease (IBD) and autoimmune diseases.

Moreover, antibiotics can interfere with the gut-brain axis, the vital communication pathway between your gut and your brain. By disrupting the gut microbiome, antibiotics can affect the production of neurotransmitters, the chemical messengers that your brain uses to regulate mood, sleep, and other functions. This can manifest as mood swings, anxiety, depression, and even cognitive impairment.

The long-term consequences of antibiotic use are still being investigated, but emerging research suggests that early-life exposure to antibiotics may have lasting effects on gut health and overall well-being. Studies have linked early antibiotic use to an increased risk of obesity, allergies, asthma, and even neurodevelopmental disorders like autism.

While antibiotics are undoubtedly valuable tools for treating bacterial infections, it's crucial to use them judiciously and only when absolutely necessary. Overuse and misuse of antibiotics can have a devastating impact on your gut microbiome, with potential consequences for your health that extend far beyond the initial infection.

Strategies for Restoring Gut Health After Antibiotics

While the collateral damage of antibiotics on your gut microbiome is undeniable, it's not a life sentence. Your gut has an incredible capacity for resilience and renewal, and with the right strategies, you can help it bounce back from the antibiotic assault and restore its healthy balance. Think of it as replanting and nurturing a garden after a devastating storm – with care and attention, it can flourish once again.

The first step in restoring your gut health after antibiotics is to replenish the beneficial bacteria that were lost during treatment. This can be achieved through a combination of dietary and supplemental interventions.

Dietary Strategies:

1. **Focus on Fiber:** Fiber is the fuel for your gut microbes. It feeds the beneficial bacteria, helping them to grow and thrive. Aim to include plenty of fiber-rich foods in your diet, such as fruits, vegetables, legumes, whole grains, nuts, and seeds.

2. **Fermented Foods:** Fermented foods like yogurt, sauerkraut, kimchi, and kefir are natural sources of probiotics, the live bacteria that can help to repopulate your gut. Aim to include a variety of fermented foods in your diet to introduce a diverse range of beneficial microbes.

3. **Prebiotics:** Prebiotics are non-digestible fibers that act as food for your gut bacteria. They selectively nourish the beneficial bacteria, helping them to outcompete harmful bacteria. Prebiotic-rich foods include onions, garlic, bananas, asparagus, and whole grains.

Supplemental Interventions:

1. **Probiotics:** Probiotic supplements can provide a concentrated dose of beneficial bacteria to help repopulate your gut. Choose a high-quality probiotic supplement that contains multiple strains of bacteria and has a high colony forming unit (CFU) count.

2. **Postbiotics:** Postbiotics are the byproducts of probiotic metabolism. They offer a range of benefits, including reducing inflammation, supporting gut barrier function, and modulating the immune system. Postbiotic supplements can be a helpful addition to your gut-healing arsenal.

3. **Other Supplements:** Certain supplements, like glutamine, zinc, and vitamin D, have been shown to support gut health and aid in recovery after antibiotic use. Consult with a healthcare professional to determine the most appropriate supplements for your individual needs.

Lifestyle Modifications:

1. **Reduce Stress:** Stress can negatively impact your gut microbiome. Find healthy ways to manage stress, such as meditation, yoga, exercise, or spending time in nature.

2. **Avoid Processed Foods and Sugar:** Processed foods and added sugar can feed harmful bacteria and hinder the growth of beneficial bacteria. Focus on whole, unprocessed foods to nourish your gut microbes.

3. **Stay Hydrated:** Drinking plenty of water is essential for

maintaining a healthy gut environment and promoting regular bowel movements.

Recovering your gut health after antibiotics takes time and patience. It's a gradual process that requires consistent effort and a holistic approach. By implementing these dietary and lifestyle strategies, you can support your gut microbiome's natural ability to heal and thrive.

Remember, your gut microbiome is a dynamic ecosystem that's constantly adapting and evolving. With the right support, it can bounce back from the challenges of antibiotic use and regain its healthy balance, contributing to your overall health and well-being.

BIRTH AND BEYOND: BUILDING A HEALTHY MICROBIOME FROM DAY ONE

The Importance of Vaginal Birth and Breastfeeding

The journey to a healthy gut microbiome begins at birth, and the first few years of life are critical for laying the foundation for a resilient and diverse gut ecosystem. The choices made during this early period, such as the mode of delivery and feeding method, can have a profound and lasting impact on a child's gut health and overall well-being.

Vaginal Birth: A Microbial Baptism

The journey through the birth canal is a transformative experience for a newborn, not just physically but also microbially. As a baby passes through the birth canal, it's exposed to a diverse array of microbes from the mother's vaginal and intestinal flora. These microbes colonize the baby's gut, skin, and respiratory tract, initiating the development of its own unique microbiome.

This microbial baptism is crucial for a healthy start in life. Studies have shown that babies born vaginally have a more diverse gut microbiome compared to those born via cesarean section. This diversity is important for training the immune system, promoting digestion, and protecting against harmful pathogens.

Babies born via cesarean section, on the other hand, miss out on this important microbial exposure. Instead, they are primarily colonized by microbes from the hospital environment and the mother's skin, which can lead to a less diverse and potentially less resilient gut microbiome. This has been linked to an increased risk of allergies, asthma, obesity, and other health problems later in life.

Breastfeeding: Nurturing the Gut Microbiome

Breast milk is nature's perfect food, providing not only essential nutrients for growth and development but also a rich source of prebiotics and probiotics that nourish and shape the infant's gut microbiome. Prebiotics, like human milk oligosaccharides (HMOs), act as food for beneficial bacteria, while probiotics, like bifidobacteria, directly colonize the gut and help to establish a healthy microbial community.

Breastfeeding has been shown to promote the growth of beneficial bacteria like bifidobacteria, which are associated with a reduced risk of infections, allergies, and chronic diseases. These bacteria help to strengthen the gut barrier, prevent the growth of harmful pathogens, and modulate the immune system.

Breast milk also contains immune factors, like antibodies and lactoferrin, that protect the infant from infections and support the development of a healthy immune system. These immune factors work in synergy with the gut microbiome, creating a powerful defense against pathogens.

Studies have shown that breastfed infants have a lower risk of developing allergies, asthma, obesity, type 1 diabetes, and other chronic diseases compared to formula-fed infants. This protective effect is thought to be due in part to the influence of breast milk on the gut microbiome.

While breastfeeding is the ideal way to nourish and shape a baby's gut microbiome, it's important to note that not all mothers can or choose to breastfeed. In these cases, formula feeding can provide essential nutrients for growth and development, and some formulas are now supplemented with prebiotics and probiotics to mimic the benefits of breast milk.

The early years of life are a critical window for shaping the gut microbiome, and the choices made during this period can have a lasting impact on health and well-being. By prioritizing vaginal birth and breastfeeding, we can give our children the best possible start in life, setting the stage for a healthy and thriving gut microbiome.

Early Life Influences on Lifelong Gut Health

The gut microbiome's journey doesn't end at birth or with the transition from breast milk to solid foods. The first few years of a child's life are a critical period for the continued development and maturation of their gut microbiome. The experiences and exposures during this time can have a profound and lasting impact on their gut health and overall well-being throughout their lives.

Diet:

As a baby transitions from breast milk or formula to solid foods, their gut microbiome undergoes significant changes. The introduction of new foods, especially those rich in fiber, can help to diversify the gut microbiome and promote the growth of beneficial bacteria. A diet rich in fruits, vegetables, whole grains, and legumes provides a variety of nutrients and fibers that nourish different types of gut microbes, fostering a balanced and resilient ecosystem.

On the other hand, a diet high in processed foods, sugary drinks, and unhealthy fats can negatively impact the gut microbiome, promoting the growth of harmful bacteria and disrupting the delicate balance of the gut ecosystem. This can lead to digestive problems, inflammation, and an increased risk of chronic diseases later in life.

Antibiotics:

While antibiotics are sometimes necessary to treat infections, their use in early life can have unintended consequences for the gut microbiome. Antibiotics can wipe out both harmful and beneficial bacteria, leading to a less diverse and potentially less resilient gut microbiome. This disruption has been linked to an increased risk of allergies, asthma, obesity, and other health problems.

It's important to use antibiotics judiciously in young children and only when absolutely necessary. If antibiotics are prescribed, consider supplementing with probiotics to help restore the balance of gut bacteria.

Environmental Exposures:

Early life exposure to environmental factors, such as pets, siblings, and daycare attendance, can influence the development of the gut microbiome. Exposure to a diverse range of microbes in the environment can help to train the immune system and promote a healthy gut microbiome.

However, excessive hygiene practices, like overuse of antibacterial soaps and disinfectants, can limit a child's exposure to beneficial microbes, potentially hindering the development of a diverse gut microbiome. It's important to strike a balance between hygiene and exposure to environmental microbes to promote a healthy gut ecosystem.

Stress:

Stress can have a significant impact on gut health at any age, but it's especially important to consider the impact of stress on young children. Stressful events, like illness, family conflict, or starting school, can disrupt the gut microbiome and increase the risk of digestive problems and other health issues.

Creating a nurturing and supportive environment for young children can help to minimize the impact of stress on their gut health. Encouraging healthy coping mechanisms, like exercise, relaxation techniques, and spending time in nature, can also help to promote a healthy gut-brain connection.

The early years of life are a critical period for shaping the gut microbiome, and the choices we make during this time can have lifelong consequences for our children's health. By understanding the factors that influence the development of the gut microbiome, we can make informed decisions that promote a healthy gut ecosystem and set the stage for a lifetime of well-being.

THE GUT-SKIN CONNECTION:
A CLEAR REFLECTION

How Gut Health Impacts Acne, Eczema, and More

Have you ever noticed a connection between your gut health and the condition of your skin? Perhaps a bout of bloating coincides with a breakout, or a flare-up of digestive issues leaves your complexion looking dull and lackluster. This isn't just a coincidence; it's a clear reflection of the gut-skin axis, a fascinating interplay between your gut microbiome and your skin health.

Your gut and your skin might seem like worlds apart, but they're actually intimately connected. This connection is mediated by a complex network of signals, including hormones, immune cells, and inflammatory molecules. When your gut microbiome is out of balance, it can trigger a cascade of events that affect your skin health, leading to a variety of skin problems, including acne, eczema, psoriasis, and rosacea.

One key player in this gut-skin connection is inflammation. When your gut microbiome is disrupted, it can trigger inflammation throughout your body, including your skin. This inflammation can manifest as redness, swelling, itching, and other skin irritations. In conditions like acne, inflammation can clog pores and lead to breakouts. In eczema, it can cause dry, itchy patches of skin.

Another factor is gut permeability, also known as "leaky gut." When your gut lining becomes compromised, it allows harmful substances, like toxins and microbes, to leak into your bloodstream. These substances can travel to your skin, triggering inflammation and contributing to skin problems.

Your gut microbiome also plays a role in regulating your immune system, which is essential for maintaining healthy skin. When your gut microbiome is out of balance, it can disrupt the balance of immune cells, leading to an overactive immune response that can manifest as skin inflammation and irritation.

For example, studies have shown that people with eczema often have an imbalanced gut microbiome, with lower levels of beneficial bacteria like bifidobacteria and lactobacilli. These bacteria help to regulate the immune system and reduce inflammation, and their absence can contribute to eczema flare-ups.

Similarly, research suggests that an imbalanced gut microbiome may play a role in the development of acne. Certain gut bacteria can produce substances that trigger inflammation and sebum production, two key factors in acne formation.

But it's not just about the bad bacteria; the good bacteria in your gut also play a crucial role in skin health. They produce short-chain fatty acids (SCFAs), which have anti-inflammatory properties and can help to soothe and heal irritated skin. They also produce vitamins and other nutrients that are essential for skin health, such as vitamin B12, which is involved in skin cell growth and repair.

By understanding the gut-skin connection, we can gain valuable insights into how to improve our skin health from the inside out. Nurturing a healthy gut microbiome through diet, lifestyle, and targeted interventions may offer a promising approach to preventing and treating a variety of skin problems.

Nutritional Strategies for a Radiant Complexion

Your skin is a reflection of your inner health, and a radiant complexion often starts from within – specifically, in your gut. By nourishing your gut microbiome with the right nutrients, you can promote a clear, healthy, and glowing skin. Think of it as feeding your skin from the inside out, providing the essential building blocks for a vibrant complexion.

Here are some key nutritional strategies for a radiant complexion, rooted in gut health:

1. **Embrace the Rainbow:** Fruits and vegetables are not only packed with vitamins and minerals, but they're also rich in antioxidants, which help protect your skin from damage caused by free radicals. Aim to fill your plate with a variety of colorful produce, including leafy greens, berries, citrus fruits, and cruciferous vegetables like broccoli and cauliflower.

2. **Fiber Up:** Fiber is essential for a healthy gut microbiome. It feeds the beneficial bacteria in your gut, helping them to thrive and produce short-chain fatty acids (SCFAs), which have anti-inflammatory properties that can benefit your skin. Aim to include plenty of fiber-rich foods in your diet, such as whole grains, legumes, fruits, and vegetables.

3. **Ferment for Your Skin:** Fermented foods, like yogurt, sauerkraut, kimchi, and kefir, are natural sources of probiotics, the live bacteria that can help to balance and diversify your gut microbiome. A healthy gut microbiome is crucial for skin health, as it can help to reduce inflammation, improve gut barrier function, and regulate the immune system.

4. **Omega-3s for Glow:** Omega-3 fatty acids are essential fats that have anti-inflammatory properties and can help to improve skin hydration and elasticity. You can find omega-3s in fatty fish like salmon, mackerel, and

sardines, as well as in flaxseeds, chia seeds, and walnuts.

5. **Hydration is Key:** Drinking plenty of water is essential for healthy skin. Water helps to flush out toxins, transport nutrients to your skin cells, and maintain skin hydration and elasticity. Aim to drink at least eight glasses of water per day.

6. **Limit Inflammatory Foods:** Certain foods, like processed foods, sugary drinks, and unhealthy fats, can trigger inflammation in your body, including your skin. Limit these foods and focus on whole, unprocessed foods to promote a healthy gut and clear skin.

7. **Consider Supplements:** While a healthy diet is the foundation for a radiant complexion, certain supplements can also be helpful. Probiotics, prebiotics, and postbiotics can support a healthy gut microbiome, while supplements like zinc, vitamin C, and collagen can provide additional benefits for your skin.

Remember, skin health is a journey, not a destination. It takes time and consistent effort to see results. By nourishing your gut microbiome with the right nutrients and adopting a healthy lifestyle, you can promote a clear, healthy, and glowing skin that reflects your inner well-being.

GUT INSTINCTS AND HEART HEALTH: AN UNEXPECTED DUO

The Gut-Heart Axis: Exploring the Connection

Your gut and your heart may seem like unlikely partners, but emerging research is revealing a surprising connection between these two seemingly disparate organs. This connection, known as the gut-heart axis, suggests that the health of your gut microbiome can significantly impact your cardiovascular well-being. It's a fascinating example of how seemingly unrelated systems in the body can be intricately linked, and how a healthy gut can pave the way for a healthy heart.

The gut-heart axis is a two-way street, with communication flowing in both directions. Your gut microbes can influence your heart health through various mechanisms, including:

1. **Metabolism of Dietary Nutrients:** Your gut microbes play a crucial role in how your body processes the food you eat. They break down dietary fiber into short-chain fatty acids (SCFAs), which have been shown to have beneficial effects on blood pressure, cholesterol levels, and inflammation - all key factors in heart health.

2. **Production of Trimethylamine N-oxide (TMAO):** Certain gut microbes can convert choline, a nutrient found in foods like eggs and red meat, into a compound called TMAO. Elevated TMAO levels have been linked to an increased risk of atherosclerosis, the buildup of plaque in the arteries that can lead to heart attacks and strokes.

3. **Regulation of Blood Pressure:** Gut microbes can influence blood pressure by modulating the production of nitric oxide, a molecule that helps to relax blood vessels and improve blood flow. An imbalance in gut bacteria can lead to reduced nitric oxide production, potentially contributing to high blood pressure.

4. **Influence on Inflammation:** Chronic inflammation is a key driver of cardiovascular disease. Gut microbes can either promote or dampen inflammation throughout your body, including in your arteries. A healthy gut microbiome, with a balance of beneficial bacteria, can help to reduce inflammation and protect your heart.

Conversely, your heart health can also impact your gut microbiome. Conditions like heart failure and high blood pressure can alter blood flow to the gut, affecting the composition and diversity of your gut microbes. This, in turn, can further exacerbate cardiovascular problems, creating a vicious cycle.

Understanding the gut-heart axis opens up new possibilities for preventing and managing heart disease. By nurturing a healthy gut microbiome, we may be able to reduce the risk of cardiovascular problems and improve outcomes for those already living with heart conditions. This can be achieved through dietary interventions, probiotic supplements, and even novel therapies like fecal microbiota transplants, which involve transferring healthy gut microbes from a donor to a recipient.

The gut-heart connection is a rapidly evolving field of research, with new discoveries constantly emerging. It's a testament to the interconnectedness of our bodies and the importance of a holistic approach to health. By recognizing the gut as a key player in cardiovascular well-being, we can develop innovative strategies to promote heart health and reduce the burden of this widespread and often deadly disease.

Microbiome-Friendly Diets for Cardiovascular Wellness

Your gut microbiome isn't just a passive bystander in your heart health journey; it's an active participant, influencing your risk of cardiovascular disease and your overall well-being. By nourishing your gut with the right foods, you can foster a healthy microbiome that supports a strong and resilient cardiovascular system. Think of it as feeding your heart through your gut, providing it with the nutrients and microbial support it needs to thrive.

A microbiome-friendly diet for cardiovascular wellness isn't about deprivation or restriction; it's about embracing whole, unprocessed foods that nourish both your body and your gut bacteria. It's a way of eating that emphasizes diversity, balance, and pleasure, while promoting optimal heart health.

Here are some key principles of a microbiome-friendly diet for cardiovascular wellness:

1. **Fiber is Your Friend:** Fiber is the fuel for your gut microbes. It feeds the beneficial bacteria, helping them to produce short-chain fatty acids (SCFAs) that have been shown to reduce inflammation, lower blood pressure, and improve cholesterol levels. Aim to include plenty of fiber-rich foods in your diet, such as fruits, vegetables, legumes, whole grains, nuts, and seeds.

2. **Ferment for Your Heart:** Fermented foods like yogurt, sauerkraut, kimchi, and kefir are natural sources of probiotics, the live bacteria that can help to balance and diversify your gut microbiome. A healthy gut microbiome is associated with a reduced risk of cardiovascular disease.

3. **Mediterranean Inspiration:** The Mediterranean diet, rich in fruits, vegetables, whole grains, legumes, fish, and olive oil, has long been associated with a reduced risk of heart disease. This diet pattern is naturally microbiome-friendly, providing a variety of nutrients and fibers that nourish beneficial gut bacteria.

4. **Limit Red Meat and Processed Foods:** Red meat, especially processed meats like bacon and sausages, have been linked to an increased risk of heart disease. These foods can also disrupt the gut microbiome, promoting the growth of harmful bacteria that produce TMAO, a compound associated with atherosclerosis. Limit your intake of red meat and processed foods, and opt for lean protein sources like fish, poultry, beans, and lentils instead.

5. **Healthy Fats for a Healthy Heart:** Not all fats are created equal. Saturated and trans fats, found in fried foods, processed snacks, and fatty cuts of meat, can raise cholesterol levels and increase the risk of heart disease. Unsaturated fats, on the other hand, found in olive oil, avocados, nuts, and fatty fish, can lower cholesterol levels and protect your heart.

6. **Plant Power:** A plant-based diet, rich in fruits, vegetables, whole grains, and legumes, is naturally microbiome-friendly and heart-healthy. Plant-based foods provide a wealth of nutrients and fiber that nourish beneficial gut bacteria, while also reducing the intake of saturated fat and cholesterol.

7. **Mindful Eating:** It's not just about what you eat, but also how you eat. Mindful eating, which involves paying attention to your hunger and fullness cues, savoring

your food, and eating without distractions, can help you make healthier choices and avoid overeating.

A microbiome-friendly diet isn't a fad or a quick fix; it's a sustainable way of eating that nourishes your body and your gut, setting the stage for a healthy heart and a long, vibrant life. By embracing whole, unprocessed foods, prioritizing fiber and fermented foods, and limiting unhealthy fats and processed foods, you can cultivate a thriving gut microbiome that supports your cardiovascular well-being.

Remember, your gut and your heart are partners in health. By nourishing your gut with the right foods, you're not just feeding your microbes; you're also feeding your heart and paving the way for a healthier, happier future.

GUT BUGS AND HORMONES: A DELICATE BALANCE

The Microbiome's Role in Thyroid, Estrogen, and More

Imagine your gut as a bustling factory, producing not just digestive enzymes but also a wide range of hormones and hormone-like substances. These gut-derived hormones play a crucial role in regulating various bodily functions, from metabolism and appetite to mood and sleep. But who's running this factory? Surprisingly, it's not just your endocrine glands, but also the trillions of microbes residing in your gut.

The gut microbiome, the vast community of microbes in your digestive tract, is a powerful influencer of your endocrine system, the network of glands that produce and regulate hormones. These microbes can produce hormones themselves, influence the production of hormones by your glands, and even modulate how your body responds to hormones.

This intricate interplay between your gut microbes and your hormones is essential for maintaining a delicate balance within your body. When this balance is disrupted, it can lead to a range of hormonal imbalances, with far-reaching consequences for your health.

One key example is the thyroid gland, a butterfly-shaped gland in your neck that produces hormones essential for regulating metabolism, energy levels, and growth. Gut microbes play a role in the conversion of inactive thyroid hormone (T4) to its active form (T3), which is necessary for proper thyroid function. An imbalance in gut bacteria can disrupt this conversion, potentially contributing to hypothyroidism, a condition characterized by low thyroid hormone levels and symptoms like fatigue, weight gain, and depression.

Another example is estrogen, a hormone that plays a key role in female reproductive health. Gut microbes can influence estrogen levels by producing an enzyme called beta-glucuronidase, which reactivates estrogen that has been processed by the liver. An overgrowth of certain bacteria can lead to elevated beta-glucuronidase levels, potentially contributing to estrogen dominance, a condition associated with irregular periods, mood swings, and an increased risk of certain cancers.

Gut microbes can also influence other hormones, such as cortisol (the stress hormone), insulin (the blood sugar-regulating hormone), and serotonin (the "happy hormone"). An imbalance in gut bacteria can disrupt the production or function of these hormones, contributing to a range of health problems, from anxiety and depression to insulin resistance and diabetes.

The gut-hormone connection is a complex and dynamic interplay, with ongoing research uncovering new layers of its influence on our health. While the exact mechanisms are still being elucidated, the evidence suggests that the gut microbiome plays a significant role in shaping our hormonal balance and overall well-being.

By understanding this connection, we can gain valuable insights into how to optimize our hormonal health. Nurturing a healthy gut microbiome through diet, lifestyle, and targeted interventions may offer a promising avenue for preventing and treating hormonal imbalances and their associated health problems.

Gut Health Strategies for Hormonal Harmony

Understanding the intricate connection between your gut microbes and your hormones is empowering. It means you have the potential to influence your hormonal health by nurturing your gut microbiome. But how exactly can you do that? It starts with embracing a gut-friendly lifestyle that includes dietary changes, targeted interventions, and mindful stress management.

Dietary Strategies:

1. Feed Your Microbes: A healthy gut microbiome thrives on a diverse diet rich in fiber. Fiber acts as food for your beneficial gut bacteria, promoting their growth and activity. Aim to include plenty of fiber-rich foods in your diet, such as fruits, vegetables, legumes, whole grains, nuts, and seeds.

2. Ferment for Hormone Balance: Fermented foods like yogurt, sauerkraut, kimchi, and kefir are natural sources of probiotics, the live bacteria that can help to balance your gut microbiome. Studies have shown that certain probiotic strains can influence hormone levels, such as reducing cortisol (the stress hormone) and improving estrogen metabolism.

3. Cruciferous Veggies for Estrogen Detox: Cruciferous vegetables like broccoli, cauliflower, kale, and Brussels sprouts contain compounds that support healthy estrogen metabolism. These compounds help to eliminate excess estrogen from your body, potentially reducing the risk of estrogen-related conditions.

4. Limit Sugar and Processed Foods: Sugar and processed foods can disrupt your gut microbiome and contribute to hormonal imbalances. These foods can feed harmful bacteria and yeast, leading to overgrowth and inflammation, which can interfere with hormone production and function.

5. Prioritize Healthy Fats: Healthy fats, like those found in olive oil, avocados, nuts, and seeds, are essential for hormone production and balance. They provide

the building blocks for hormones and help to regulate inflammation, which can impact hormonal health.

Targeted Interventions:

1. Probiotics: If you're experiencing hormonal imbalances, specific probiotic strains may be helpful. Lactobacillus and Bifidobacterium strains have been shown to influence estrogen metabolism, reduce cortisol levels, and improve thyroid function. Consult with a healthcare professional to determine the most appropriate probiotic strains for your individual needs.

2. Prebiotics: Prebiotics, like inulin and fructooligosaccharides (FOS), nourish the beneficial bacteria in your gut, promoting their growth and activity. This can help to create a balanced gut microbiome that supports hormonal health.

3. Herbal Remedies: Certain herbs, like ashwagandha, maca root, and chasteberry, have traditionally been used to support hormonal balance. These herbs may work by modulating hormone levels, reducing stress, and supporting the gut microbiome. Consult with a healthcare professional before taking any herbal supplements.

Stress Management:

Chronic stress can wreak havoc on your hormonal balance. It can elevate cortisol levels, disrupt other hormone production, and contribute to gut dysbiosis. Finding healthy ways to manage stress, like meditation, yoga, deep breathing exercises, or spending time in nature, can help to restore hormonal harmony and promote a healthy gut microbiome.

Remember, gut health and hormonal health are interconnected. By nourishing your gut with a healthy diet, incorporating targeted interventions like probiotics and prebiotics, and managing stress, you can create a harmonious environment for your hormones to thrive.

The gut-hormone connection is a fascinating and rapidly evolving field of research, and understanding this connection can empower you to take charge of your hormonal health and overall well-being.

MICROBIOME AND AGING: NURTURING YOUR INNER ECOSYSTEM

Age-Related Changes in the Gut

Just as our bodies undergo changes as we age, so too does our gut microbiome, the vast community of microbes residing in our digestive tract. This internal ecosystem, which plays a crucial role in our health and well-being, isn't immune to the passage of time. Understanding the age-related changes in the gut microbiome can empower us to take proactive steps to nurture this ecosystem and promote healthy aging.

As we grow older, our gut microbiome tends to become less diverse. This means we have fewer types of bacteria, and the relative abundance of different species can shift. While some beneficial bacteria may decline, others, including opportunistic pathogens, may increase. This loss of diversity can weaken the gut's resilience, making it more susceptible to imbalances and disruptions.

One of the most significant changes is a decrease in the abundance of Bifidobacteria. These beneficial bacteria play a key role in maintaining gut barrier integrity, regulating the immune system, and producing essential vitamins and short-chain fatty acids. A decline in Bifidobacteria can lead to increased gut permeability ("leaky gut"), inflammation, and a compromised immune response, making us more vulnerable to infections and chronic diseases.

Another common age-related change is an increase in the abundance of potentially harmful bacteria, such as Enterobacteriaceae. These bacteria can produce toxins and trigger inflammation in the gut, contributing to digestive problems and other health issues.

The aging process also affects the production of digestive enzymes and stomach acid. These substances are essential for breaking down food and absorbing nutrients, and their decline can lead to indigestion, bloating, and nutrient deficiencies.

The gut lining, which acts as a barrier between the gut contents and the bloodstream, can also become thinner and more permeable with age. This can allow harmful substances, like toxins and microbes, to leak into the bloodstream, triggering inflammation and potentially contributing to chronic diseases.

Several factors contribute to these age-related changes in the gut microbiome. Our diet, which tends to become less diverse and fiber-rich as we age, can influence the types of bacteria that thrive in our gut. Medications, especially antibiotics, can also disrupt the gut microbiome, and their use often increases with age. Lifestyle factors, like physical activity levels and stress, can also influence gut health, and these factors often change as we get older.

But it's important to remember that these changes are not inevitable. While aging may naturally lead to some shifts in the gut microbiome, we can take proactive steps to support a healthy gut ecosystem throughout our lives. By adopting a gut-friendly diet, incorporating probiotics and prebiotics, staying active, managing stress, and avoiding unnecessary antibiotics, we can nurture our gut microbiome and promote healthy aging.

Understanding the age-related changes in the gut microbiome is just the first step. In the next part, we'll explore practical strategies for maintaining a healthy gut as we age, including dietary recommendations, supplement options, and lifestyle modifications. By taking care of our gut microbiome, we're not just supporting our digestive health; we're also promoting our overall well-being and longevity.

Probiotics and Diet for Healthy Aging

While age-related changes in the gut microbiome are a natural part of life, they don't have to dictate your health destiny. By proactively nurturing your gut microbiome, you can support healthy aging and potentially mitigate some of the negative effects associated with an aging gut. Let's delve into two powerful tools in your gut health arsenal: probiotics and a gut-friendly diet.

Probiotics: Your Gut's Best Friends

Probiotics are live microorganisms that, when consumed in adequate amounts, confer a health benefit on the host. In simpler terms, they're the "good" bacteria that can help to restore balance and diversity to your gut microbiome. As we age, our gut microbiome tends to lose diversity and beneficial bacteria, making probiotics an especially important tool for seniors.

Research suggests that probiotics may offer a range of benefits for aging individuals, including:

- **Improved digestion:** Probiotics can help to break down food, reduce gas and bloating, and promote regular bowel movements. This can be particularly beneficial for older adults who may experience digestive problems due to decreased enzyme production and slower gut motility.
- **Enhanced immune function:** Probiotics can help to stimulate the immune system and reduce inflammation, which can help to protect against infections and chronic diseases. This is especially important for older adults, who may have a weakened immune system due to age-related changes.
- **Increased nutrient absorption:** Probiotics can help to improve the absorption of certain nutrients, such as calcium and vitamin B12, which are essential for bone health and cognitive function.
- **Reduced risk of chronic diseases:** Studies suggest that

probiotics may help to reduce the risk of chronic diseases like heart disease, type 2 diabetes, and certain types of cancer.

When choosing a probiotic for healthy aging, look for a high-quality supplement that contains multiple strains of bacteria, particularly those that have been shown to be beneficial for older adults, such as Bifidobacterium and Lactobacillus strains. Consult with a healthcare professional to determine the most appropriate probiotic for your individual needs.

Diet: The Foundation for a Healthy Gut

What you eat plays a crucial role in shaping your gut microbiome, and this becomes even more important as you age. A gut-friendly diet can help to nourish beneficial bacteria, reduce inflammation, and support optimal gut function.

Here are some key dietary recommendations for healthy aging:

- **Fiber-Rich Foods:** Fiber is the fuel for your gut microbes. It feeds the beneficial bacteria, helping them to thrive and produce short-chain fatty acids (SCFAs), which have numerous health benefits. Aim to include plenty of fiber-rich foods in your diet, such as fruits, vegetables, legumes, whole grains, nuts, and seeds.
- **Fermented Foods:** Fermented foods like yogurt, sauerkraut, kimchi, and kefir are natural sources of probiotics, the live bacteria that can help to balance your gut microbiome. Aim to include a variety of fermented foods in your diet to introduce a diverse range of beneficial microbes.
- **Prebiotics:** Prebiotics are non-digestible fibers that act as food for your gut bacteria. They selectively nourish the beneficial bacteria, helping them to outcompete harmful bacteria. Prebiotic-rich foods include onions, garlic, bananas, asparagus, and whole grains.
- **Limit Processed Foods, Sugar, and Unhealthy Fats:** These foods can disrupt your gut microbiome and contribute to inflammation. Focus on whole, unprocessed foods to nourish

your gut microbes.

- **Stay Hydrated:** Drinking plenty of water is essential for maintaining a healthy gut environment and promoting regular bowel movements.

By incorporating these dietary and lifestyle strategies, you can nurture your gut microbiome and support healthy aging. Remember, it's never too late to start taking care of your gut health.

THE MICROBIOME AND THE MIND: BEYOND THE GUT-BRAIN AXIS

Gut Bacteria and Neurodegenerative Diseases

While the gut-brain connection has been well-established, with clear links between gut health and mental well-being, emerging research is now revealing a potential connection between the gut microbiome and neurodegenerative diseases. This growing body of evidence suggests that the trillions of microbes residing in our gut may play a role in the development and progression of conditions like Alzheimer's disease, Parkinson's disease, and multiple sclerosis (MS).

It might seem surprising that gut bacteria, located far from the brain, could influence such complex neurological disorders. But remember, the gut and the brain are in constant communication through the gut-brain axis, a bi-directional highway of signals that travel through nerves, hormones, and the immune system.

This connection is not just about influencing mood and behavior; it also involves the immune system and inflammation, both of which are implicated in neurodegenerative diseases. An imbalanced gut microbiome can trigger inflammation throughout the body, including the brain, and contribute to the neurodegeneration that characterizes these diseases.

For example, studies have shown that people with Alzheimer's disease often have a less diverse gut microbiome compared to healthy individuals. They tend to have lower levels of beneficial bacteria that produce anti-inflammatory substances, and higher levels of bacteria that produce pro-inflammatory molecules. This imbalance can lead to chronic inflammation in the brain, contributing to the accumulation of amyloid plaques and tau tangles, hallmarks of Alzheimer's disease.

In Parkinson's disease, a neurodegenerative disorder characterized by tremors and movement difficulties, gut dysbiosis has also been observed. Some studies suggest that certain gut bacteria may trigger the misfolding of alpha-synuclein, a protein that accumulates in the brains of people with Parkinson's. This misfolding can lead to the formation of Lewy bodies, another hallmark of the disease.

Multiple sclerosis (MS), an autoimmune disease that affects the central nervous system, has also been linked to gut microbiome imbalances. Research suggests that certain gut bacteria may trigger an autoimmune response that damages the protective myelin sheath around nerve fibers, leading to the neurological symptoms of MS.

While the exact mechanisms linking the gut microbiome to neurodegenerative diseases are still being elucidated, the emerging evidence suggests that gut bacteria may play a role in the development, progression, and potentially even prevention of these devastating conditions.

By understanding this connection, we can explore new avenues for treatment and prevention. Probiotic supplements, dietary interventions, and fecal microbiota transplants are just some of the potential strategies being investigated for their ability to modulate the gut microbiome and potentially slow or even reverse the progression of neurodegenerative diseases.

The microbiome and the mind are intricately connected, and the gut-brain axis is far more complex than we once thought. As research continues to uncover the links between gut health and neurological disorders, we're gaining valuable insights into how we can harness the power of our gut microbiome to protect our brains and promote lifelong cognitive health.

Exploring the Gut-Brain Connection in Autism

Autism spectrum disorder (ASD) is a complex neurodevelopmental condition characterized by challenges with social interaction, communication, and repetitive behaviors. While the exact causes of ASD remain unclear, emerging research is shedding light on a potential connection between gut health and autism. This connection is not a simple cause-and-effect relationship, but rather a complex interplay between the gut microbiome, the immune system, and the brain.

Children with ASD often experience gastrointestinal (GI) problems, such as constipation, diarrhea, and abdominal pain, at a higher rate than neurotypical children. These GI issues have led researchers to investigate the role of the gut microbiome in autism. Studies have shown that children with ASD often have a less diverse gut microbiome compared to neurotypical children. They may also have an overgrowth of certain harmful bacteria and a deficiency of beneficial bacteria.

This gut dysbiosis could contribute to autism in several ways:

1. Gut-Brain Axis Disruption: The gut and the brain are in constant communication through the gut-brain axis. An imbalanced gut microbiome can disrupt this communication, affecting the development and function of the brain. For example, certain gut bacteria can produce neurotransmitters and other molecules that influence brain development and behavior.

2. Inflammation: Gut dysbiosis can trigger inflammation throughout the body, including the brain. This inflammation can disrupt brain development and function, potentially contributing to the neurological

symptoms of autism.

3. Immune Dysregulation: The gut microbiome plays a crucial role in educating and regulating the immune system. An imbalanced gut microbiome can lead to immune dysregulation, which has been implicated in autism. Studies have shown that children with ASD often have abnormal immune responses, and some researchers believe that these immune abnormalities may be triggered by gut dysbiosis.

4. Leaky Gut: An imbalanced gut microbiome can weaken the gut barrier, leading to a condition known as "leaky gut." This allows harmful substances, like toxins and microbes, to leak into the bloodstream and potentially reach the brain, where they can trigger inflammation and damage.

While the gut-brain connection in autism is still an active area of research, the emerging evidence suggests that the gut microbiome may be a promising target for interventions. Some studies have shown that probiotic supplements, dietary interventions, and fecal microbiota transplants may improve GI symptoms and even some behavioral symptoms in children with ASD.

It's important to note that the gut microbiome is just one piece of the complex puzzle of autism. Genetics, environmental factors, and other biological processes also play a role. However, by understanding the gut-brain connection in autism, we can open up new avenues for research and potential treatments for this complex condition.

If you're a parent of a child with ASD, it's important to work with a healthcare professional to address any GI issues your child may be experiencing. Dietary interventions, such as a gluten-free or casein-free diet, or probiotic supplements, may be helpful in some cases. However, it's crucial to consult with a healthcare professional before starting any new treatment for your child.

The gut-brain connection in autism is a rapidly evolving field of research, and we can expect to see many more exciting discoveries in the years to come. By exploring this connection, we may be able to develop new therapies and interventions that can improve the lives of individuals with ASD and their families.

THE GUT FEELING REVOLUTION:
THE FUTURE OF MEDICINE

Fecal Microbiota Transplants (FMT): A New Frontier in Gut Health

Imagine a treatment that sounds straight out of science fiction: transplanting poop from a healthy person into the gut of someone with a serious illness. It might sound gross, but this revolutionary procedure, known as fecal microbiota transplantation (FMT), is emerging as a game-changer in the world of medicine, particularly in the realm of gut health.

FMT involves transferring a carefully screened and processed stool sample from a healthy donor into the recipient's gut, usually through a colonoscopy, endoscopy, or capsules. This infusion of healthy microbes can repopulate the recipient's gut microbiome, restoring balance and diversity, and potentially reversing a range of gut-related disorders.

It's a bit like pressing the reset button on a malfunctioning computer. When your gut microbiome is out of whack due to disease, medication, or lifestyle factors, it can lead to a host of health problems. FMT provides a fresh start, introducing a healthy and diverse community of microbes that can outcompete harmful bacteria, reduce inflammation, and restore gut function.

FMT has shown remarkable success in treating Clostridium difficile (C. diff) infection, a debilitating and potentially life-threatening bacterial infection that causes severe diarrhea and inflammation of the colon. C. diff often occurs after antibiotic use, which can disrupt the gut microbiome and allow C. diff to flourish. While antibiotics can treat the initial infection, they often fail to prevent recurrence. FMT, on the other hand, has a success rate of over 90% in resolving recurrent C. diff infections, making it a life-saving treatment for many patients.

But the potential of FMT extends far beyond C. diff. Researchers are exploring its use in a variety of other gut-related disorders, including inflammatory bowel disease (IBD), irritable bowel syndrome (IBS), and even obesity and metabolic syndrome. Studies have shown promising results in some cases, with FMT leading to improvements in symptoms, reduced inflammation, and even remission of disease.

The gut-brain axis, the bidirectional communication pathway between the gut and the brain, also opens up exciting possibilities for FMT. Researchers are investigating its potential in treating neurological and psychiatric conditions, such as Parkinson's disease, multiple sclerosis, and autism. While research is still in its early stages, the results so far are promising, suggesting that FMT could one day revolutionize the way we treat these complex conditions.

FMT is not without its risks and challenges. The screening process for donors is rigorous to ensure the safety of the transplanted material. There's also the potential for unintended consequences, as we're still learning about the complex interactions between gut microbes and the human body. However, the potential benefits of FMT are undeniable, and it's rapidly emerging as a powerful tool in the fight against gut-related disorders.

FMT represents a paradigm shift in medicine, moving away from the traditional "one-size-fits-all" approach to treatment and embracing a more personalized and holistic approach that recognizes the crucial role of the gut microbiome in our health. It's a testament to the interconnectedness of our bodies and the power of harnessing the natural healing potential of our gut microbes.

Personalized Medicine Based on

Gut Microbiome Analysis

Imagine a world where medical treatments are no longer one-size-fits-all, but instead, tailored precisely to your individual needs. This is the promise of personalized medicine, and the gut microbiome is playing a starring role in this emerging revolution. By analyzing the unique composition of your gut microbes, scientists and healthcare providers are gaining valuable insights into your health risks, disease susceptibility, and treatment response. This personalized approach to medicine could revolutionize the way we prevent, diagnose, and treat a wide range of diseases.

Your gut microbiome is like a fingerprint, unique to you and shaped by a combination of genetics, diet, lifestyle, and environmental factors. This microbial community plays a crucial role in your health, influencing everything from digestion and immunity to mental health and hormone balance. By analyzing the specific microbes present in your gut, we can gain a deeper understanding of your individual health profile.

Gut microbiome analysis, also known as microbiome sequencing or profiling, involves collecting a stool sample and analyzing the DNA of the microbes present. This provides a detailed snapshot of your gut microbiome, revealing the types and abundance of different bacteria, viruses, fungi, and other microbes residing in your gut.

This information can be used in several ways:

1. Disease Risk Assessment: Certain gut microbiome profiles have been associated with an increased risk of various diseases, such as inflammatory bowel disease, obesity, type 2 diabetes, and even certain types of cancer. By analyzing your gut microbiome, healthcare providers can identify potential risk factors and develop personalized prevention strategies.

2. Diagnosis: Gut microbiome analysis can also aid in the diagnosis of certain conditions. For example, an overgrowth of certain bacteria can be a sign of small intestinal bacterial overgrowth (SIBO), while a lack of specific bacteria may indicate inflammatory bowel disease.

3. Treatment Optimization: Your gut microbiome can also influence how your body responds to medications. For example, certain gut microbes can metabolize drugs, affecting their efficacy and side effects. By analyzing your gut microbiome, healthcare providers can tailor your treatment plan to optimize its effectiveness and minimize adverse reactions.

4. Personalized Nutrition: Your gut microbes play a crucial role in how your body processes food and extracts nutrients. Microbiome analysis can identify potential food sensitivities and intolerances, allowing you to personalize your diet for optimal digestion and nutrient absorption.

5. Monitoring and Tracking: Your gut microbiome is not static; it's constantly changing and evolving in response to diet, lifestyle, and other factors. Regular microbiome analysis can track these changes over time, allowing you to monitor your gut health and make adjustments as needed to maintain a healthy and balanced microbiome.

The Gut Feeling Revolution: The Future of Medicine

Personalized medicine based on gut microbiome analysis is still in its early stages, but it holds immense promise for the future of healthcare. As research continues to uncover the links between the gut microbiome and various diseases, we can expect to see more sophisticated and accurate microbiome-based diagnostics and treatments.

This personalized approach to medicine could revolutionize the way we prevent, diagnose, and treat a wide range of conditions, from digestive disorders and metabolic diseases to autoimmune disorders and even mental health conditions. It could also lead to more targeted and effective treatments, reducing the risk of side effects and improving patient outcomes.

The gut feeling revolution is just beginning, and it's an exciting time to be exploring the potential of this new frontier in medicine. By understanding the role of the gut microbiome in our health and embracing personalized medicine, we can unlock a new era of health and well-being.

THE GUT HEALTH TOOLKIT: TESTS, TREATMENTS, AND THERAPIES

Understanding Gut Health Testing Options

Imagine your gut as a complex machine, with numerous gears and levers working together to maintain optimal function. Just like any machine, your gut can malfunction from time to time, leading to digestive problems, inflammation, and other health issues. But how do you know what's going on inside your gut and what steps you need to take to restore its health? This is where gut health testing comes in.

Gut health testing is like a diagnostic tool that allows you to peek inside your gut and uncover the secrets of your microbiome. It can provide valuable insights into the composition of your gut microbes, identify potential imbalances, and pinpoint the root causes of your symptoms. Armed with this information, you and your healthcare provider can develop a personalized plan to restore your gut health and optimize your overall well-being.

But with so many different gut health tests available, how do you know which one is right for you? Let's break down the most common types of tests and their benefits:

1. **Stool Tests:**
- **Microbiome Analysis (Stool Test):** This comprehensive test analyzes the DNA of the microbes in your stool sample, providing a detailed snapshot of your gut microbiome. It can identify the types and abundance of different bacteria, fungi, and other microbes, revealing potential imbalances and risk factors for various diseases.

- **Comprehensive Stool Analysis:** This test goes beyond just identifying microbes. It also assesses markers of inflammation, digestion, and gut barrier function, providing a more complete picture of your gut health.

- **Parasitology Test:** This test checks for the presence of parasites in your stool, which can cause a range of digestive problems.

2. **Breath Tests:**

- **Hydrogen Breath Test (HBT):** This test measures the amount of hydrogen in your breath after you consume a specific type of sugar. It can help to diagnose small intestinal bacterial overgrowth (SIBO), a condition where bacteria from your large intestine overgrows in your small intestine, causing digestive problems.

- **Lactose Breath Test:** This test measures the amount of hydrogen in your breath after you consume lactose, the sugar found in milk and dairy products. It can help to diagnose lactose intolerance, a condition where your body lacks the enzyme lactase, which is needed to digest lactose.

3. **Blood Tests:**

- **Food Sensitivity Testing:** This test measures your immune system's reaction to different foods, identifying potential food sensitivities. However, the accuracy and reliability of these tests are controversial, and more research is needed to validate their effectiveness.

- **C-Reactive Protein (CRP):** This test measures the level of CRP, a protein that indicates inflammation in your body. Elevated CRP levels can be a sign of various conditions, including gut inflammation.

4. **Other Tests:**

- **Gastric Emptying Study:** This test measures how quickly food leaves your stomach. It can help to diagnose delayed gastric emptying, a condition where your stomach takes longer than usual to empty.

- **Endoscopy and Colonoscopy:** These invasive procedures allow doctors to directly visualize your gut lining and take tissue samples for analysis. They're typically used to diagnose more serious conditions like inflammatory bowel disease (IBD) or colon cancer.

Choosing the right gut health test depends on your individual needs and symptoms. If you're experiencing digestive problems, a comprehensive stool analysis or microbiome analysis might be helpful. If you suspect a food sensitivity, a food sensitivity test or elimination diet could be a good option. And if you're experiencing more severe symptoms, your doctor may recommend an endoscopy or colonoscopy.

It's important to consult with a healthcare professional to discuss your symptoms and determine the most appropriate testing options for you. They can help you interpret the test results and develop a personalized plan to restore your gut health.

Navigating Probiotics, Prebiotics, and Other Therapies

With the increasing awareness of the gut microbiome's importance for overall health, a wide array of treatments and therapies have emerged, promising to restore balance and improve gut function. From probiotics and prebiotics to herbal remedies and dietary changes, the options can seem overwhelming. Let's break down these various approaches and explore how they can be integrated into a comprehensive gut health plan.

Probiotics: Replenishing the Good Guys

Probiotics are live microorganisms that, when consumed in adequate amounts, confer a health benefit on the host. In simpler terms, they're the "good" bacteria that can help to repopulate your gut with beneficial microbes and restore a healthy balance. Probiotics can be found in fermented foods like yogurt, sauerkraut, and kimchi, as well as in dietary supplements.

Different strains of probiotics offer different benefits, so it's important to choose the right ones for your specific needs. For example, Lactobacillus rhamnosus GG has been shown to be effective in preventing and treating diarrhea, while Bifidobacterium lactis may help reduce anxiety and stress. Consult with a healthcare professional to determine the most appropriate probiotic strains for your individual needs.

Prebiotics: Feeding the Good Guys

Prebiotics are non-digestible fibers that act as food for your gut bacteria. They selectively nourish the beneficial bacteria, helping them to thrive and outcompete harmful bacteria. Prebiotics are found in foods like onions, garlic, bananas, asparagus, and whole grains.

Incorporating prebiotic-rich foods into your diet can help to create a thriving environment for your gut microbes. You can also find prebiotic supplements, which can be a convenient way to boost your intake of these beneficial fibers.

Postbiotics: The Power of Byproducts

Postbiotics are the byproducts of probiotic metabolism, the substances that probiotics produce as they break down food and interact with your gut environment. These byproducts have a range of beneficial effects, including reducing inflammation, supporting gut barrier function, and modulating the immune system.

While research on postbiotics is still in its early stages, they show promise as a potential therapeutic tool for gut health. Postbiotic supplements are becoming increasingly available, but you can also find postbiotics naturally in fermented foods like sauerkraut and kimchi.

Dietary Interventions:

The food you eat plays a crucial role in shaping your gut microbiome. A diet rich in fiber, fermented foods, and whole grains can promote a healthy and diverse gut ecosystem. Conversely, a diet high in processed foods, sugar, and unhealthy fats can disrupt your gut microbiome and contribute to a range of health problems.

Eliminating or reducing trigger foods, such as gluten, dairy, or certain types of sugar, can also be helpful for some individuals with specific food sensitivities or intolerances. Working with a healthcare professional or registered dietitian can help you identify potential trigger foods and develop a personalized elimination diet.

Other Therapies:

- Fecal Microbiota Transplantation (FMT): As discussed in Chapter 15, FMT is a revolutionary treatment that involves transplanting healthy gut microbes from a donor to a recipient. It has shown remarkable success in treating C. diff infection and is being explored for other gut-related disorders.

- Herbal Remedies: Certain herbs, like peppermint, ginger, and chamomile, have traditionally been used to soothe digestive discomfort and promote gut health. However, it's important to consult with a healthcare professional before taking any herbal supplements, as they can interact with medications and may not be appropriate for everyone.

- Stress Management: Chronic stress can negatively impact

your gut microbiome. Finding healthy ways to manage stress, such as meditation, yoga, exercise, or spending time in nature, can help to restore gut balance and improve overall well-being.

The gut health toolkit is vast and varied, offering a range of options for restoring and maintaining a healthy gut microbiome. By understanding these different approaches and working with a healthcare professional, you can develop a personalized plan that addresses your specific needs and goals, leading to a healthier gut and a happier you.

NOURISHING YOUR MICROBIOME: A CULINARY ADVENTURE

Fermented Foods: The Gut's Best Friends

Embark on a culinary journey to nourish your gut microbiome, and you'll find yourself exploring a world of vibrant flavors and textures. Fermented foods, often considered ancient culinary treasures, are making a comeback in the modern kitchen as we rediscover their remarkable benefits for gut health. These tangy, effervescent delights not only tantalize our taste buds but also provide a powerful boost to our internal ecosystem of microbes.

What are Fermented Foods?

Fermentation is a natural process where microorganisms like bacteria and yeasts break down sugars and starches in food, transforming them into acids, gases, and alcohol. This process not only preserves food but also creates unique flavors and textures, while increasing the bioavailability of nutrients. Think of fermentation as a culinary alchemy that transforms ordinary ingredients into gut-loving superfoods.

The Gut-Friendly Power of Fermentation

Fermented foods are teeming with probiotics, the live bacteria that can help to replenish and diversify your gut microbiome. These beneficial microbes play a crucial role in maintaining a healthy gut environment, supporting digestion, boosting immunity, and even influencing your mood and mental health.

But the benefits of fermented foods go beyond just probiotics. Fermentation also produces prebiotics, the non-digestible fibers that act as food for your gut bacteria, as well as postbiotics, the beneficial byproducts of probiotic metabolism. This trifecta of gut-friendly compounds makes fermented foods a nutritional powerhouse for your microbiome.

A World of Fermented Flavors

Fermented foods come in a dazzling array of flavors and textures, from tangy sauerkraut and kimchi to creamy yogurt and kefir, to fizzy kombucha and sourdough bread. Here are some popular fermented foods to explore:

- **Yogurt:** A creamy dairy product made by fermenting milk with live bacteria cultures. Choose plain yogurt with live and active cultures for maximum gut health benefits.
- **Sauerkraut:** A tangy condiment made from fermented cabbage. It's rich in probiotics and vitamin C, which can boost your immune system.
- **Kimchi:** A spicy Korean side dish made from fermented vegetables, typically cabbage, radishes, and scallions. It's packed with probiotics, vitamins, and minerals.
- **Kefir:** A tangy fermented milk drink similar to yogurt but with a thinner consistency. It's rich in probiotics and calcium, making it a great choice for gut and bone health.
- **Kombucha:** A fizzy fermented tea drink made with a SCOBY (symbiotic culture of bacteria and yeast). It's a good source of probiotics and antioxidants.
- **Miso:** A savory paste made from fermented soybeans. It's a good source of probiotics, protein, and minerals.
- **Tempeh:** A fermented soybean cake with a firm texture and nutty flavor. It's a good source of probiotics, protein, and fiber.
- **Sourdough bread:** Made with a sourdough starter, a fermented mixture of flour and water. It's easier to digest than regular bread and may have a lower glycemic index.

Incorporating fermented foods into your diet is a delicious and effective way to nourish your gut microbiome. Start by adding small amounts to your meals and gradually increase your intake as your gut adjusts. You can enjoy them as a side dish, a condiment, or even incorporate them into your main courses for a flavor and probiotic boost.

Building a Gut-Friendly Diet: Recipes and Tips

While fermented foods are a delicious and convenient way to nourish your gut microbiome, they're just one piece of the puzzle. A holistic approach to gut health involves creating a balanced and diverse diet that provides a wide range of nutrients and fibers to support the diverse community of microbes residing in your gut.

Here are some key principles for building a gut-friendly diet:

1. Embrace the Rainbow: Fruits and vegetables are not only packed with vitamins, minerals, and antioxidants, but they're also rich in prebiotics, the non-digestible fibers that feed your beneficial gut bacteria. Aim to fill your plate with a variety of colorful produce, including leafy greens, berries, citrus fruits, and cruciferous vegetables like broccoli and cauliflower.

2. Prioritize Whole Grains: Whole grains like oats, quinoa, brown rice, and whole-wheat bread are excellent sources of fiber, which is essential for a healthy gut microbiome. They also provide complex carbohydrates, which are slowly digested and provide sustained energy, unlike refined grains, which can spike blood sugar levels and disrupt gut bacteria.

3. Legumes for Gut Health: Legumes like lentils, beans, chickpeas, and peas are nutritional powerhouses, packed with fiber, protein, and resistant starch, a type of carbohydrate that acts as a prebiotic and promotes the growth of beneficial bacteria. Incorporate legumes into your meals as a meat substitute, add them to salads, or

use them to make hearty soups and stews.

4. Nuts and Seeds for Microbiome Diversity: Nuts and seeds are a good source of healthy fats, protein, and fiber. They also contain polyphenols, plant compounds with antioxidant and anti-inflammatory properties that can benefit your gut microbes. Snack on a handful of nuts or seeds, sprinkle them on your salads or yogurt, or blend them into smoothies for a gut-friendly boost.

5. Limit Processed Foods and Sugar: Processed foods and added sugar can disrupt your gut microbiome and contribute to inflammation. These foods often contain artificial ingredients, preservatives, and unhealthy fats that can harm your gut microbes. Instead, focus on whole, unprocessed foods that nourish your body and your gut.

6. Mindful Eating: It's not just about what you eat, but also how you eat. Mindful eating, which involves paying attention to your hunger and fullness cues, savoring your food, and eating without distractions, can help you make healthier choices and avoid overeating. Chewing your food thoroughly and eating slowly can also aid in digestion and promote gut health.

Gut-Friendly Recipes:

Here are a few simple and delicious recipes that incorporate gut-friendly ingredients:

- **Overnight Oats:** Combine rolled oats, milk (dairy or plant-based), chia seeds, yogurt, and your favorite fruits and nuts in a jar. Let it sit overnight in the refrigerator, and you'll have a delicious and gut-healthy breakfast ready in the morning.

- **Lentil Soup:** Sauté onions, carrots, celery, and garlic in olive oil. Add lentils, vegetable broth, diced tomatoes, and your favorite spices. Simmer until the lentils are tender, and enjoy a hearty and fiber-rich soup that's good for your gut.

- **Quinoa Salad with Roasted Vegetables:** Roast your favorite vegetables like broccoli, cauliflower, Brussels sprouts, and sweet potatoes. Cook quinoa according to package directions. Combine the roasted vegetables, quinoa, chopped herbs, nuts, seeds, and a vinaigrette dressing made with olive oil, lemon juice, and herbs. Enjoy a colorful and nutritious salad packed with gut-friendly ingredients.

Building a gut-friendly diet is a journey of exploration and discovery. Experiment with different ingredients, flavors, and recipes to find what works best for you and your gut microbiome. Remember, a healthy gut is a happy gut, and a happy gut can lead to a healthier and happier you.

THE DIRTY TRUTH: ENVIRONMENTAL TOXINS AND GUT HEALTH

How Pesticides, Heavy Metals, and Plastics Harm the Gut

Imagine your gut as a delicate ecosystem, a thriving community of microbes working tirelessly to keep you healthy. But this ecosystem is constantly under threat from a barrage of environmental toxins that we encounter daily in our food, water, and air. These toxins, like pesticides, heavy metals, and plastics, can wreak havoc on your gut microbiome, disrupting its delicate balance and potentially leading to a host of health problems.

Pesticides: The Silent Disruptors

Pesticides are chemicals used to kill pests that damage crops and livestock. While they may protect our food supply, they can also harm our gut microbes. Many pesticides are designed to disrupt the nervous system of insects, but they can also affect the nervous system of our gut bacteria. This can lead to imbalances in the gut microbiome, reducing the diversity of beneficial bacteria and creating an environment where harmful bacteria can thrive.

Studies have linked pesticide exposure to a variety of gut-related problems, including leaky gut syndrome, inflammatory bowel disease (IBD), and even changes in gut motility. Pesticides can also disrupt the gut-brain axis, the vital communication pathway between your gut and your brain, potentially contributing to mood disorders and cognitive problems.

Heavy Metals: The Toxic Burden

Heavy metals like lead, mercury, arsenic, and cadmium are naturally occurring elements that can contaminate our food and water supply through industrial pollution, mining, and other human activities. These toxins can accumulate in our bodies over time, and the gut is a major site of heavy metal absorption.

Once inside the gut, heavy metals can disrupt the gut microbiome, killing beneficial bacteria and creating an environment where harmful bacteria can flourish. This can lead to inflammation, oxidative stress, and damage to the gut lining, potentially contributing to a range of health problems, from digestive issues to neurological disorders.

Plastics: The Unseen Invaders

Plastics are ubiquitous in our modern world, from food packaging and water bottles to toys and personal care products. But these seemingly harmless materials contain a cocktail of chemicals, including phthalates and bisphenol A (BPA), which can leach into our food and drinks and ultimately end up in our gut.

These plastic-derived chemicals are known endocrine disruptors, meaning they can interfere with our hormones and disrupt the delicate balance of our endocrine system. This can have a wide range of health effects, including reproductive problems, developmental issues, and even an increased risk of certain cancers.

In addition to their endocrine-disrupting effects, plastic-derived chemicals can also harm our gut microbiome. Studies have shown that these chemicals can alter the composition and diversity of gut bacteria, potentially contributing to inflammation, gut barrier dysfunction, and other health problems.

The Dirty Truth

The truth is, we're constantly exposed to a wide range of environmental toxins that can harm our gut health. While it's impossible to avoid all exposure, we can take steps to minimize our exposure and protect our gut microbiome.

Protecting Your Microbiome from Environmental Threats

While the prevalence of environmental toxins may seem daunting, there are practical steps you can take to minimize your exposure and protect your precious gut microbiome. Think of it as fortifying your gut's defenses, creating a resilient ecosystem that can withstand the onslaught of environmental assaults.

Dietary Strategies:

1. Choose Organic: Opt for organic produce whenever possible to reduce your exposure to pesticides. While organic food can be more expensive, prioritize the "Dirty Dozen," the fruits and vegetables with the highest pesticide residues, like strawberries, spinach, and grapes.

2. Filter Your Water: Invest in a high-quality water filter to remove heavy metals, chlorine, and other contaminants from your drinking water. Consider using a filter for your shower water as well, as your skin can absorb toxins during bathing.

3. Cook at Home: By preparing your own meals, you have more control over the ingredients and can reduce your exposure to processed foods, which often contain added sugars, unhealthy fats, and artificial ingredients that can disrupt your gut microbiome.

4. Choose Sustainable Seafood: Certain fish, like tuna and swordfish, can contain high levels of mercury, a heavy metal that can harm your gut and your overall health. Choose smaller fish like sardines, anchovies, and herring, which are lower in mercury and rich in omega-3

fatty acids, which are beneficial for gut health.

5. Limit Plastic Exposure: Reduce your exposure to plastic-derived chemicals by choosing glass or stainless steel containers for food storage and drinking water. Avoid heating food in plastic containers, as heat can accelerate the leaching of chemicals. Opt for natural personal care products that are free of phthalates and parabens.

Lifestyle Modifications:

1. Support Detoxification: Your body has a natural detoxification system that helps to eliminate toxins. You can support this system by eating a diet rich in cruciferous vegetables (like broccoli, cauliflower, and kale), drinking plenty of water, and sweating through exercise or sauna use.

2. Manage Stress: Chronic stress can weaken your gut barrier and make you more susceptible to the effects of environmental toxins. Find healthy ways to manage stress, such as meditation, yoga, deep breathing exercises, or spending time in nature.

3. Get Enough Sleep: Adequate sleep is essential for overall health, including gut health. Aim for 7-8 hours of sleep per night to support your body's natural repair and detoxification processes.

4. Exercise Regularly: Exercise can help to improve gut motility, reduce inflammation, and boost the diversity of your gut microbiome. Aim for at least 30 minutes of moderate-intensity exercise most days of the week.

Supplements:

1. Probiotics and Prebiotics: Probiotic and prebiotic supplements can help to restore and maintain a healthy gut microbiome, which is crucial for protecting against the harmful effects of environmental toxins. Consult with a healthcare professional to determine the most appropriate supplements for your individual needs.

2. Glutathione: Glutathione is a powerful antioxidant that plays a key role in detoxification. Supplementing with glutathione or its precursors, like N-acetylcysteine (NAC), may help to protect your gut from oxidative stress caused by environmental toxins.

3. Activated Charcoal: Activated charcoal is a porous substance that can bind to toxins and help to remove them from your body. It can be taken as a supplement or used topically to detoxify the skin.

Protecting your gut microbiome from environmental toxins is an ongoing process that requires vigilance and a holistic approach. By making informed choices about your diet, lifestyle, and supplement use, you can create a resilient gut ecosystem that can withstand the challenges of modern life and support your overall health and well-being.

THE MICROBIOME MAKEOVER: A STEP-BY-STEP GUIDE

Assessing Your Gut Health: Where to Start

Embarking on a journey to improve your gut health can feel like navigating uncharted territory. With so much information and conflicting advice, it's easy to feel overwhelmed and unsure of where to start. But just like any makeover, transforming your gut health begins with an assessment – a thorough evaluation of your current state to identify areas that need attention and create a personalized plan for improvement.

Think of it like a home renovation project. Before you start knocking down walls or choosing paint colors, you need to assess the existing structure, identify any problems, and create a blueprint for your renovation. Similarly, before you embark on a gut health makeover, you need to assess your current gut health, pinpoint any imbalances or issues, and develop a tailored plan to restore balance and optimize your gut function.

So, how do you assess your gut health? There are several approaches you can take, each offering unique insights into your gut's inner workings:

1. Symptom Checklist:

One of the simplest and most accessible ways to assess your gut health is to pay attention to your body's signals. Your gut is constantly communicating with you, and your symptoms can provide valuable clues about its health. Common gut-related symptoms include:

- Digestive issues: Bloating, gas, constipation, diarrhea, heartburn, indigestion

- Fatigue and low energy
- Skin problems: Acne, eczema, rosacea
- Mood issues: Anxiety, depression, brain fog
- Food sensitivities or intolerances
- Autoimmune conditions

While these symptoms can be caused by a variety of factors, their frequent or persistent presence may indicate an underlying gut health issue. Keeping a symptom diary can help you track your symptoms and identify any patterns or triggers.

2. Dietary Evaluation:

Your diet plays a crucial role in shaping your gut microbiome. A diet high in processed foods, sugar, and unhealthy fats can disrupt your gut microbes and contribute to inflammation, while a diet rich in fiber, fermented foods, and whole grains can nourish beneficial bacteria and promote a healthy gut environment.

Evaluating your current diet can help you identify areas for improvement. Are you getting enough fiber? Are you eating a variety of fruits, vegetables, and whole grains? Are you consuming fermented foods regularly? By honestly assessing your dietary habits, you can pinpoint any areas that need attention and make adjustments to support your gut health.

3. Gut Health Testing:

While observing your symptoms and evaluating your diet can provide valuable insights, gut health testing can offer a more in-depth look at your gut microbiome. These tests, which typically involve analyzing a stool sample, can identify the types and abundance of microbes in your gut, reveal potential imbalances, and pinpoint any underlying infections or inflammation.

Several types of gut health tests are available, including:

- Microbiome analysis: This comprehensive test analyzes the DNA of the microbes in your stool, providing a detailed snapshot of your gut microbiome.

- Comprehensive stool analysis: This test goes beyond identifying microbes, also assessing markers of inflammation, digestion, and gut barrier function.
- Food sensitivity testing: This test measures your immune system's reaction to different foods, identifying potential food sensitivities.

Consult with a healthcare professional to determine which gut health test is most appropriate for you. They can help you interpret the results and develop a personalized plan to address any imbalances or issues that may be present.

Assessing your gut health is the crucial first step in your microbiome makeover journey. By taking the time to understand your gut's unique needs and challenges, you can create a targeted and effective plan to restore balance, optimize function, and ultimately improve your overall health and well-being.

A Personalized Plan for Optimal Gut Health

Armed with insights from your gut health assessment, it's time to craft a personalized plan to transform your gut microbiome and optimize your well-being. Think of it as a tailor-made wardrobe for your gut, where each piece is carefully chosen to fit your unique needs and style. This plan isn't about strict rules or deprivation; it's about making sustainable changes that nourish your gut and fit seamlessly into your lifestyle.

1. Nourish Your Microbes with a Gut-Friendly Diet:

Your diet is the cornerstone of gut health. By making simple yet impactful changes, you can create a microbiome-friendly environment that fosters the growth of beneficial bacteria and reduces inflammation.

- Embrace Fiber: Aim for at least 30 grams of fiber per day. This includes a variety of fruits, vegetables, legumes, whole grains, nuts, and seeds. Gradually increase your fiber intake to allow your gut to adjust, and drink plenty of water to prevent constipation.

- Ferment for Flavor and Function: Incorporate fermented foods into your diet regularly. Yogurt, sauerkraut, kimchi, kefir, kombucha, and other fermented delights are packed with probiotics that can replenish and diversify your gut microbiome.

- Prebiotic Power: Include prebiotic-rich foods in your meals and snacks. Onions, garlic, bananas, asparagus, and whole grains are just a few examples of foods that feed your beneficial gut bacteria.

- Limit Processed Foods and Sugar: These foods can disrupt your gut microbiome and contribute to inflammation. Instead, focus on whole, unprocessed foods that nourish your body and your gut.

2. Supplement Strategically:

Supplements can be a helpful addition to your gut health plan, but they shouldn't replace a healthy diet. Consult with a healthcare professional to determine which supplements are right for you.

- Probiotics: Choose a high-quality probiotic supplement that contains multiple strains of beneficial bacteria and has a high colony forming unit (CFU) count.

- Prebiotics: If your diet lacks prebiotic-rich foods, consider taking a prebiotic supplement to nourish your gut bacteria.

- Other Supplements: Certain supplements, like glutamine, zinc, and omega-3 fatty acids, may also be beneficial for gut health. However, consult with a healthcare professional before starting any new supplements.

3. Lifestyle Modifications:

Your lifestyle choices can significantly impact your gut health. By making simple adjustments, you can create an environment that supports a healthy microbiome.

- Manage Stress: Chronic stress can wreak havoc on your gut microbiome. Find healthy ways to manage stress, such as meditation, yoga, deep breathing exercises, or spending time in nature.

- Prioritize Sleep: Adequate sleep is essential for gut health and overall well-being. Aim for 7-8 hours of sleep per night to allow your body to rest and repair.

- Exercise Regularly: Exercise can improve gut motility, reduce inflammation, and boost the diversity of your gut microbiome. Aim for at least 30 minutes of moderate-intensity exercise most days of the week.

- Stay Hydrated: Drinking plenty of water is essential for maintaining a healthy gut environment and promoting regular bowel movements.

4. Personalized Touches:

Your gut microbiome is unique, and your plan should reflect that. Consider your individual needs, preferences, and lifestyle when making dietary and lifestyle changes.

- Food Sensitivities: If you have any food sensitivities or intolerances, be sure to eliminate or reduce those foods from your diet.

- Medical Conditions: If you have any underlying medical conditions, consult with your healthcare provider before making any significant changes to your diet or lifestyle.

- Budget and Lifestyle: Choose gut-friendly foods that fit

your budget and lifestyle. There are plenty of delicious and affordable options available, so you don't have to break the bank to nourish your gut.

By following these steps and creating a personalized plan, you can embark on a microbiome makeover journey that transforms your gut health and overall well-being. Remember, it's a marathon, not a sprint. Be patient, persistent, and kind to yourself along the way.

THE GUT FEELING PRESCRIPTION: YOUR PATH TO WELLNESS

Empowering Yourself with Knowledge

The journey to optimal gut health isn't just about following a set of rules or adopting a specific diet. It's about understanding the intricate workings of your gut microbiome and its profound impact on your overall well-being. It's about empowering yourself with knowledge, so you can make informed decisions about your health and create a lifestyle that supports a thriving gut ecosystem.

Think of it like learning a new language. At first, it may seem overwhelming, with unfamiliar terms and complex concepts. But as you delve deeper, you begin to understand the nuances, the connections, and the underlying principles. You gain confidence in your ability to communicate and navigate this new world. Similarly, as you learn more about your gut microbiome, you gain a deeper understanding of its language, its needs, and its responses. This knowledge empowers you to make choices that support its health and, in turn, your overall well-being.

Here are some key areas of knowledge that can empower you on your gut health journey:

1. The Microbiome Basics: Understanding the composition and diversity of your gut microbiome, the different types of microbes, and their roles in your body is fundamental. This knowledge lays the groundwork for understanding how your gut microbiome impacts your health and how you can influence it through diet and

lifestyle.

2. Gut-Body Connection: The gut microbiome is not just a digestive organ; it's a complex ecosystem that interacts with virtually every system in your body. It influences your immune system, your brain, your hormones, and even your skin. Understanding these connections can help you appreciate the far-reaching impact of your gut health on your overall well-being.

3. Diet and the Microbiome: Your diet plays a crucial role in shaping your gut microbiome. Learn about the foods that nourish beneficial bacteria, like fiber, fermented foods, and prebiotics. Understand how processed foods, sugar, and unhealthy fats can disrupt your gut microbes. This knowledge empowers you to make informed food choices that support a healthy gut.

4. Gut Health Testing: Explore the different types of gut health tests available, such as microbiome analysis, comprehensive stool analysis, and breath tests. Understand their benefits and limitations, and consult with a healthcare professional to determine which tests are right for you. These tests can provide valuable insights into your gut health and guide your treatment decisions.

5. Lifestyle Factors: Your lifestyle choices, such as sleep, exercise, and stress management, can significantly impact your gut health. Learn about the lifestyle factors that promote a healthy gut microbiome and those that can disrupt it. This knowledge allows you to make positive changes to your lifestyle that support your gut health.

6. Treatments and Therapies: Explore the various

treatments and therapies available for gut health, such as probiotics, prebiotics, postbiotics, dietary interventions, and fecal microbiota transplants (FMT). Understand how these therapies work, their potential benefits, and their risks. This knowledge allows you to make informed decisions about your treatment options in consultation with your healthcare provider.

7. Gut Health Resources: Seek out reliable and evidence-based information about gut health. There are many books, websites, and experts that can provide you with valuable information and support. Stay informed about the latest research and developments in the field of gut health, so you can make the best decisions for your well-being.

Empowering yourself with knowledge is the first step towards taking control of your gut health. By understanding the intricate workings of your gut microbiome and its impact on your health, you can make informed decisions about your diet, lifestyle, and treatment choices. This knowledge is not just power; it's the key to unlocking a healthier, happier, and more vibrant you.

Building a Lifestyle for Lifelong Gut Health

Empowering yourself with knowledge about your gut microbiome is only the first step in your journey toward optimal well-being. To truly reap the benefits of a healthy gut, you need to integrate that knowledge into your daily life, creating a lifestyle that supports and nourishes your internal ecosystem. Think of it as cultivating a thriving garden within you, where the seeds of well-being can blossom and flourish.

Here's how you can build a lifestyle for lifelong gut health:

1. Nourish with Food: Your diet is the most direct way to influence your gut microbiome. Embrace a whole-food,

plant-based approach that prioritizes fiber, diversity, and fermented foods. Fill your plate with colorful fruits and vegetables, whole grains, legumes, nuts, and seeds. Experiment with fermented delights like yogurt, sauerkraut, kimchi, and kombucha. Limit processed foods, sugar, and unhealthy fats, which can disrupt the delicate balance of your gut microbes.

2. Cultivate Mindful Eating Habits: Slow down and savor each bite. Pay attention to your hunger and fullness cues. Eat without distractions, like phones or screens. Chew your food thoroughly to aid digestion. Mindful eating not only enhances the enjoyment of your meals but also promotes better digestion and nutrient absorption.

3. Move Your Body: Regular exercise is not just good for your heart and muscles; it also benefits your gut microbiome. Studies have shown that exercise can increase the diversity of gut bacteria and reduce inflammation. Find activities you enjoy, whether it's dancing, swimming, hiking, or simply taking a brisk walk. Aim for at least 30 minutes of moderate-intensity exercise most days of the week.

4. Manage Stress: Chronic stress can wreak havoc on your gut health by disrupting the delicate balance of your gut microbiome and triggering inflammation. Find healthy ways to manage stress, such as meditation, yoga, deep breathing exercises, spending time in nature, or pursuing hobbies you enjoy. Prioritize self-care and make time for relaxation and rejuvenation.

5. Prioritize Sleep: Sleep is a time for your body to rest and repair, and your gut microbiome is no exception. During sleep, your gut microbes undergo important processes

that support their growth and function. Aim for 7-8 hours of quality sleep each night to allow your gut microbiome to flourish.

6. Supplement Wisely: While a healthy diet and lifestyle are the foundation of gut health, supplements like probiotics and prebiotics can be helpful additions. Probiotics can replenish your gut with beneficial bacteria, while prebiotics provide nourishment for these microbes. Consult with a healthcare professional to determine the right supplements for your individual needs.

7. Stay Informed: The field of gut health is rapidly evolving, with new research and discoveries emerging constantly. Stay up-to-date on the latest findings by reading books, articles, and blogs from reputable sources. Consider joining online communities or forums where you can connect with others on a gut health journey.

8. Listen to Your Gut: Your gut is constantly sending you signals about its health. Pay attention to your body's whispers, whether it's bloating, gas, constipation, or other digestive discomfort. These signals may indicate an imbalance or issue that needs attention. Don't hesitate to seek guidance from a healthcare professional if you have concerns about your gut health.

Building a lifestyle for lifelong gut health is an ongoing process. It's not about perfection but about progress. By embracing these principles and making sustainable changes, you can create a harmonious relationship with your gut microbiome, supporting your overall health and well-being for years to come. Remember, your gut feeling is more than just intuition; it's a compass guiding you towards a healthier and happier life.

9 798325 594106